Orthopedic Anesthesiology

Editors

PHILIPP LIRK
KAMEN VLASSAKOV

ANESTHESIOLOGY CLINICS

www.anesthesiology.theclinics.com

Consulting Editor
LEE A. FLEISHER

September 2022 • Volume 40 • Number 3

ELSEVIER

1600 John F. Kennedy Boulevard • Suite 1800 • Philadelphia, Pennsylvania, 19103-2899

http://www.theclinics.com

ANESTHESIOLOGY CLINICS Volume 40, Number 3
September 2022 ISSN 1932-2275, ISBN-13: 978-0-323-91957-9

Editor: Joanna Collett
Developmental Editor: Arlene Campos

Anesthesiology Clinics (ISSN 1932-2275) is published quarterly by Elsevier Inc., 360 Park Avenue South, New York, NY 10010-1710. Months of issue are March, June, September, and December. Periodicals postage paid at New York, NY and at additional mailing offices. Subscription prices are $100.00 per year (US student/resident), $375.00 per year (US individuals), $464.00 per year (Canadian individuals), $986.00 per year (US institutions), $1016.00 per year (Canadian institutions), $100.00 per year (Canadian student/resident), $225.00 per year (foreign student/resident), $498.00 per year (foreign individuals), and $1016.00 per year (foreign institutions). To receive student and resident rate, orders must be accompanied by name of affiliated institution, date of term, and the *signature* of program/residency coordinator on institutions letterhead. Orders will be billed at individual rate until proof of status is received. Foreign air speed delivery is included in all *Clinics'* subscription prices. All prices are subject to change without notice. POSTMASTER: Send address changes to *Anesthesiology Clinics,* Elsevier Health Sciences Division, Subscription Customer Service, 3251 Riverport Lane, Maryland Heights, MO 63043. Customer Service (orders, claims, online, change of address): Elsevier Health Sciences Division, Subscription Customer Service, 3251 Riverport Lane, Maryland Heights, MO 63043. **Tel:1-800-654-2452 (U.S. and Canada); 314-447-8871 (outside U.S. and Canada). Fax: 314-447-8029. E-mail: journalscustomerservice-usa@elsevier.com (for print support); journalsonlinesupport-usa@elsevier.com (for online support).**

Reprints. For copies of 100 or more of articles in this publication, please contact the Commercial Reprints Department, Elsevier Inc., 360 Park Avenue South, New York, NY 10010-1710. Tel.: 212-633-3874; Fax: 212-633-3820; E-mail: reprints@elsevier.com.

Anesthesiology Clinics, is also published in Spanish by McGraw-Hill Inter-americana Editores S. A., P.O. Box 5-237, 06500 Mexico D. F., Mexico.

Anesthesiology Clinics, is covered in *MEDLINE/PubMed (Index Medicus), Current Contents/Clinical Medicine, Excerpta Medica, ISI/BIOMED,* and *Chemical Abstracts.*

Printed in the United States of America.

Contributors

CONSULTING EDITOR

LEE A. FLEISHER, MD, FACC, FAHA
Robert D. Dripps Professor and Chair of Anesthesiology and Critical Care, Professor of Medicine, Perelman School of Medicine, University of Pennsylvania, Philadelphia, Pennsylvania

EDITORS

PHILIPP LIRK, MD, MSc, PhD
Attending Anesthesiologist, Department of Anesthesiology, Perioperative and Pain Medicine, Brigham and Women's Hospital, Associate Professor, Harvard Medical School, Boston, Massachusetts, USA

KAMEN VLASSAKOV, MD, FASA
Chief, Division of Regional and Orthopedic Anesthesiology, Perioperative and Pain Medicine, Brigham and Women's Hospital; Associate Professor, Anaesthesia, Harvard Medical School; Director, Regional Anesthesiology and Acute Pain Medicine Fellowship; Department of Anesthesiology, Perioperative and Pain Medicine, Brigham and Women's Hospital, Boston, Massachusetts, USA

AUTHORS

JOSÉ A. AGUIRRE, MD, MSc
EDRA, Senior Consultant Anesthetist, Head of Ambulatory Center Europaallee, Stadtspital Zürich, Institute of Anaesthesiology, Triemli City Hospital Zürich, Balgrist Campus, Zürich, Switzerland

WALID ALRAYASHI, MD
Instructor, Harvard Medical School, Director, Home Analgesia Program, Department of Anesthesiology, Critical Care and Pain Medicine, Boston Children's Hospital, Boston, Massachusetts, USA

HELENE BELOEIL, MD, PhD
Anesthesia and Intensive Care Department, Univ Rennes, Inserm CIC 1414, COSS 1242, CHU Rennes, Rennes, France

ALAIN BORGEAT, MD
Senior Consultant, Balgrist Campus, Zurich, Switzerland; Department of Surgery, University of Illinois at Chicago, Chicago, Illinois, USA

ROLAND BRUSSEAU, MD
Assistant Professor, Harvard Medical School, Director, Pediatric Regional Anesthesia Program, Department of Anesthesiology, Critical Care and Pain Medicine, Boston Children's Hospital, Boston, Massachusetts, USA

CRISPIANA COZOWICZ, MD
Department of Anesthesiology, Critical Care and Pain Management, Hospital for Special Surgery, Weill Cornell Medical College, New York, New York, USA; Department of Anesthesiology, Perioperative Medicine and Intensive Care Medicine, Paracelsus Medical University, Salzburg, Austria

JOSEPH CRAVERO, MD
Professor, Harvard Medical School, Anesthesiologist-in-Chief, Department of Anesthesiology, Critical Care and Pain Medicine, Boston Children's Hospital, Boston, Massachusetts, USA

ANIS DIZDAREVIC, MD
Attending Physician, Department of Anesthesiology, Columbia University Irving Medical Center, New York, New York, USA

NABIL M. ELKASSABANY, MD, MSCE
Associate Professor, Department of Anesthesiology and Critical Care, Perelman School of Medicine, University of Pennsylvania, Philadelphia, Pennsylvania, USA

RODNEY A. GABRIEL, MD, MAS
Associate Professor of Anesthesiology, In Residence, University of California, San Diego, San Diego, California

PHILIPP GERNER, MD
Department of Anesthesiology, Critical Care and Pain Medicine, Massachusetts General Hospital, Harvard Medical School, Boston, Massachusetts, USA

RAJNISH K. GUPTA, MD
Professor, Department of Anesthesiology, Vanderbilt University Medical Center, Nashville, Tennessee, USA

MITCHEL B. HARRIS, MD
Massachusetts General Hospital, Boston, Massachusetts, USA

YOLANDA HUANG, MD
Attending Physician, Department of Anesthesiology, Columbia University Irving Medical Center, New York, New York, USA

BRIAN M. ILFELD, MD, MS
Professor of Anesthesiology, In Residence, University of California, San Diego, Department of Anesthesiology, La Jolla, California, USA

PHILIPP LIRK, MD, MSc, PhD
Attending Anesthesiologist, Department of Anesthesiology, Perioperative and Pain Medicine, Brigham and Women's Hospital, Associate Professor, Harvard Medical School, Boston, Massachusetts, USA

THUAN LY, MD
Massachusetts General Hospital, Boston, Massachusetts, USA

STAVROS G. MEMTSOUDIS, MD, PhD, MBA
Department of Anesthesiology, Critical Care and Pain Management, Hospital for Special Surgery, Weill Cornell Medical College, New York, New York, USA; Department of Anesthesiology, Perioperative Medicine and Intensive Care Medicine, Paracelsus Medical University, Salzburg, Austria

ARCHANA O'NEILL, MD
Department of Anesthesiology, Perioperative and Pain Medicine, Brigham and Women's Hospital, Harvard Medical School, Boston, Massachusetts, USA

CHRISTIAN PEAN, MD, MS
Brigham and Women's Hospital, Boston, Massachusetts, USA

RICHA SHARMA, MBBS
Resident Physician, Department of Anesthesiology, Columbia University Irving Medical Center, New York, New York, USA

ALEXANDER STONE, MD
Department of Anesthesiology, Perioperative and Pain Medicine, Brigham and Women's Hospital, Harvard Medical School, Boston, Massachusetts, USA; Department of Anesthesiology, Hospital for Special Surgery, New York, New York, USA

IMRÉ VAN HERREWEGHE, MD
Consultant Anesthesiologist, Department of Anesthesiology, AZ Turnhout, Turnhout, Belgium

LETITIA VAN PACHTENBEKE, MD
Anesthesia Resident, Department of Anesthesiology, Ziekenhuis Oost-Limburg, Genk, Belgium

CATHERINE VANDEPITTE, MD, PhD
Consultant Anesthesiologist, Department of Anesthesiology, Ziekenhuis Oost-Limburg, Genk, Belgium

KAMEN VLASSAKOV, MD, FASA
Chief, Division of Regional and Orthopedic Anesthesiology, Associate Professor, Anesthesia, Harvard Medical School, Director, Regional Anesthesiology and Acute Pain Medicine Fellowship, Anesthesiology, Perioperative and Pain Medicine, Brigham and Women's Hospital, Boston, Massachusetts, USA

ARVIND G. VON KEUDELL, MD, MPH
Brigham and Women's Hospital, Boston, Massachusetts, USA; Bispebjerg Hospital, Universtiy of Copenhagen, Copenhagen, København, Denmark

MICHAEL J. WEAVER, MD
Brigham and Women's Hospital, Boston, Massachusetts, USA

MORNÉ WOLMARANS, MD
EDRA, Consultant Anesthetist, Department of Anesthesia, Norfolk and Norwich University Hospital NHS Trust, Past President, Regional Anesthesia UK (RA-UK), ESRA Board Member, Norwich, United Kingdom

Contents

The body of literature concerning the influence of anesthetic type on many perioperative outcomes has grown considerably in recent years. Most studies have suggested that particularly in orthopedic patients, regional anesthesia may be associated with improved perioperative outcomes. Orthopedic trauma presents itself as a field that might benefit from increased utilization of regional techniques with the goal to improve outcomes. This narrative review concludes that, indeed, regional anesthesia seems to provide benefits for morbidity, pain control, and improved return to function in hip fracture, rib fracture, and isolated extremity fracture patients.

Patients who have perioperatively benefited from regional anesthesia frequently report moderate to severe pain when the nerve block effects fade away. Over the past years, the term "rebound pain" has been introduced, suggesting a specific pathologic process. It is debated whether significant pain on block resolution reflects a separate and distinct pathologic mechanism potentially involving proinflammatory and neurotoxic effects of local anesthetics, or is simply caused by the recovery of sensory function at a timepoint when nociceptive stimuli are still intense, and moderate to severe pain should be anticipated. In that latter case, the phenomenon referred to as rebound pain could be considered a failure of pain management providers to devise an adequate analgesia plan. Whatever the ultimate designation, management of rebound pain should be proactive, by implementing multimodal analgesia, or tailoring the blockade to the expected trajectory of postoperative pain and managing patient expectations accordingly. Until we know more about the etiology and impact of this phenomenon, the authors suggest a more neutral designation such as "pain on block resolution."

Acute compartment syndrome (ACS) is a potential orthopedic emergency
that leads, without prompt diagnosis and immediate treatment with surgical fasciotomy, to permanent disability. The role of regional anesthesia
(RA) for analgesia in patients at risk for ACS remains unjustifiably controversial. This critical review aims to improve the perception of the published
literature to answer the question, whether RA techniques actually delay or
may even help to hasten the diagnosis of ACS. According to literature, peripheral RA alone does not delay ACS diagnosis and surgical treatment.
Only in 4 clinical cases, epidural analgesia was associated with delayed
ACS diagnosis.

Orthopedic surgery procedures involving joint arthroplasty, complex
spine, long bone and pelvis procedure, and trauma and oncological cases
can be associated with a high risk of bleeding and need for blood transfusion, making efforts to optimize patient care and reduce blood loss very
important. Patient blood management programs incorporate efforts to
optimize preoperative anemia, develop transfusion protocols and restrictive hemoglobin triggers, advance surgical and anesthesia practice, and
use antifibrinolytic therapies. Perioperative management of anticoagulant
therapies, a multidisciplinary decision-making task, weighs in risks and
benefits of thromboembolic risk and surgical bleeding and is patient-
and surgery-specific.

Opioid-free anesthesia is a multimodal anesthesia aimed at avoiding the
negative impact of intraoperative opioid on patient's postoperative outcomes. It is based on the physiology of pathways involved in intraoperative
nociception. It has been shown to be feasible but the literature is still
scarce on the clinically meaningful benefits as well as on the side effects
and/or complications that might be associated with it. Moreover, most
studies involved abdominal and/or bariatric surgery. Procedure-specific
studies are lacking, especially in orthopedics.

Joint replacements are increasingly performed as outpatient surgeries.
The push toward ambulatory joint arthroplasty is driven in part by the
changing current health care economics and reimbursement models. Patients' selection and well-designed perioperative care pathways are critical
for the success of these procedures. The rate of complications after

ANESTHESIOLOGY CLINICS

FORTHCOMING ISSUES

December 2022
Vascular Anesthesia
Megan P. Kostibas and Heather K.
Hayanga, *Editors*

March 2023
**Current Topics in Critical Care for the
Anesthesiologist**
Athanasios Chalkias, Mary Jarzebowski,
and Kathryn Rosenblatt, *Editors*

September 2023
Geriatric Anesthesia
Shamsuddin Akhtar, *Editor*

RECENT ISSUES

June 2022
Total Well-being
Alison J. Brainard and Lyndsay M. Hoy,
Editors

March 2022
**Enhanced Recovery After Surgery and
Perioperative Medicine**
Michael J. Scott, Anton Krige Michael, and
Patrick William Grocott, *Editors*

December 2021
Obstetrical Anesthesia
May C.M. Pian-Smith and Rebecca D.
Minehart, *Editors*

SERIES OF RELATED INTEREST

Critical Care Clinics

Foreword

Orthopedic Anesthesiology: A Constantly Evolving Area of Perioperative Care

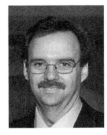

Lee A. Fleisher, MD, FACC, FAHA
Consulting Editor

Orthopedic surgery is among the most common procedures performed in individuals, particularly those at the extremes of age. This includes elective procedures as well as addressing trauma victims. Given the large number of similar procedures with an ability to standardize perioperative care, it has been an area of intense interest for the application of Enhanced Recovery after Surgery protocols as well as perioperative pain management, including regional anesthesia strategies. While these protocols have demonstrated improvement in outcomes, there are also risks that must be considered. In this issue of *Anesthesiology Clinics*, the editors have included many strategies that can both improve outcomes and potentially mitigate risks through knowledge.

In order to commission an issue on orthopedic anesthesia care, I have turned to colleagues at Harvard Medical School and the Brigham and Women's Hospital. Philipp Lirk, MD, PhD is Associate Professor of Anaesthesia. He served as Associate Editor for the *European Journal of Anaesthesiology.* Dr Lirk has worked in PROSPECT, an interdisciplinary working group affiliated with the European Society of Regional Anaesthesia and Pain Therapy, to formulate Evidence-based and Procedure-specific Acute Pain Management guidelines. Kamen Vlassakov, MD is Associate Professor

Anesthesiology Clin 40 (2022) xiii–xiv
https://doi.org/10.1016/j.anclin.2022.08.001
1932-2275/22/© 2022 Published by Elsevier Inc.

of Anaesthesia. He is Director of the Division of Regional and Orthopedic Anesthesia at the Brigham and Women's Hospital. Together, they have edited an important issue.

Lee A. Fleisher, MD, FACC, FAHA
3400 SPRUCE STREET, DULLES 680
Philadelphia, PA 19104, USA

E-mail address:
Lee.Fleisher@pennmedicine.upenn.edu

Preface

Orthopedic Anesthesiology 2022

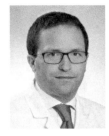 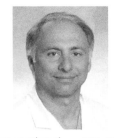

Philipp Lirk, MD, MSc, PhD   Kamen Vlassakov, MD, FASA
Editors

Orthopedic anesthesiology continues to evolve as a subspecialty practice niche with its specific challenges and progress, and in natural unison with regional anesthesiology and acute pain medicine. It is also logically intertwined with the multifaceted practice of modern orthopedic surgery in its entire scope, as well as the age- and comorbidity-specific expertise of different medical specialties, such as geriatrics, all in dynamic clinical collaborations to design, improve, and implement optimal patient care.

In this issue of *Anesthesiology Clinics*, we have tried to build upon the conversation started in 2014 (Orthopedic anesthesia. *Anesthesiol Clin.* 2014 Dec;32(4)) with updates and "deeper dives" into some of the topics relevant to clinical practice and outcomes that orthopedic anesthesiologists wake up and go to sleep with every workday.

Importantly, this project was conceived and realized under the extreme circumstances of the COVID-19 pandemic and unprecedented work force shortages, including academic human resources. We were very lucky to tap into the tremendous wealth of knowledge shared by a joint team of experts from North America and Europe that made our ambitious plan possible, despite significant setbacks and with only minor goal and scope resets.

In this issue, important up-to-date reviews of outcomes after orthopedic trauma surgery, multimodal analgesia, same-day arthroplasty surgery, pediatric regional anesthesia in orthopedic surgery, and opioid-sparing techniques are enriched by a timely review of relevant blood-conservation strategies and are further "spiced up" by an update on innovative methods to extend postoperative analgesia and discussions of controversial topics, such as rebound pain after peripheral nerve blocks, and acute compartment syndrome and regional anesthesia. And, finally, it is adorned by an opinion piece by prominent orthopedic trauma surgery colleagues, providing a glimpse into their viewpoints, biases, and appreciation of the complex multidisciplinary care for our patients.

Anesthesiology Clin 40 (2022) xv–xvi
https://doi.org/10.1016/j.anclin.2022.08.002
1932-2275/22/© 2022 Published by Elsevier Inc.

With our humility, deep respect, and best wishes to the *Anesthesiology Clinics* readership, we would also like to express our profound gratitude to our distinguished Team:

To our authors, for their selfless work and readiness to generously share unparalleled individual and collective expertise!

To our publishing production team, for their unwavering support, patience, and understanding!

To all our families, for their unconditional love and support during these many hours of "after hours" and weekend work!

Philipp Lirk, MD, MSc, PhD
Department of Anesthesiology
Perioperative and Pain Medicine
Brigham and Women's Hospital
Harvard Medical School
75 Francis Street
Boston, MA 02115, USA

39 Court Street
Dedham, MA, 02026, USA

Kamen Vlassakov, MD, FASA
Division of Regional and Orthopedic Anesthesiology
Department of Anesthesiology
Perioperative and Pain Medicine
Brigham and Women's Hospital
Harvard Medical School
75 Francis Street
Boston, MA 02115, USA

E-mail addresses:
plirk@bwh.harvard.edu (P. Lirk)
kvlassakov@bwh.harvard.edu (K. Vlassakov)

Outcomes After Orthopedic Trauma Surgery – What is the Role of the Anesthesia Choice?

Philipp Gerner, MD[a], Crispiana Cozowicz, MD[b,c],
Stavros G. Memtsoudis, MD, PhD, MBA[b,c,*]

KEYWORDS

- Orthopedic trauma • Regional anesthesia • Hip fracture • Rib fracture
- Anesthetic choice • Peripheral nerve block • Neuraxial

KEY POINTS

- For hip fracture, rib fracture, and isolated extremity fracture, regional anesthesia seems to provide outcome benefits.
- The choice between regional and general anesthesia in orthopedic trauma should take into consideration multiple factors, including injury burden and patient-specific factors.
- The role of anesthesia in orthopedic trauma continues to evolve.

INTRODUCTION

The last decade has seen an ever-growing focus on implementing regional techniques into anesthetic practice. The advent of ultrasound, the formation of specialized training programs, and improved procedure-related safety profiles, have led to an increase in understanding of how regional techniques can be used to effectively spare patients the often-significant implications of a general anesthetic, including cardiovascular and central nervous system depression.

The benefits of regional techniques seem to be related to a number of intrinsic factors. Blockade of afferent and efferent nerve function is associated with several physiologic effects that mechanistically can explain improved outcomes in clinical

[a] Department of Anesthesiology, Critical Care and Pain Medicine, Massachusetts General Hospital, Harvard Medical School, 55 Fruit Street, Boston, MA 02143, USA; [b] Department of Anesthesiology, Critical Care and Pain Management, Hospital for Special Surgery, Weill Cornell Medical College, 535 East 70th Street, New York, NY 10021, USA; [c] Department of Anesthesiology, Perioperative Medicine and Intensive Care Medicine, Paracelsus Medical University, Muellner Hauptstrasse 48, Salzburg 5020, Austria
* Corresponding author. Department of Anesthesiology, Critical Care and Pain Management, Hospital for Special Surgery, Weill Cornell Medical College, 535 East 70th Street, New York, NY 10021, USA
E-mail address: memtsoudiss@hss.edu

Anesthesiology Clin 40 (2022) 433–444
https://doi.org/10.1016/j.anclin.2022.04.001
1932-2275/22/© 2022 Elsevier Inc. All rights reserved.
anesthesiology.theclinics.com

practice. These include the suppression of the pathophysiologic cascade of the stress response to surgical stimulus via the use of neuraxial anesthesia and peripheral nerve blocks (PNBs).[1] Additionally, regional anesthesia often allows omission of airway manipulation and decreased need for systemic analgesia, permitting reduced opioid consumption and facilitating expedited recovery.[2–4] Moreover, complications related to the procedures themselves are rare.[5,6]

The body of literature concerning the influence of anesthetic type on many perioperative outcomes has grown considerably in recent years. Most studies have suggested that particularly in orthopedic patients, regional anesthesia may be associated with improved perioperative outcomes.[7,8] Of course, anesthesia for orthopedic surgery remains diverse in techniques used. The umbrella term of regional anesthesia includes many different approaches such as neuraxial, peripheral nerve blocks (PNBs), and intravenous (IV) regional techniques.

While consensus on the best approach to elective orthopedic cases such as total hip and knee arthroplasty have been published,[9] the approach to orthopedic trauma presents a challenging topic. It must be acknowledged that trauma patients represent a widely heterogeneous population requiring a diverse set of interventions. Outcomes associated with these procedures will, therefore, often depend on the severity of trauma and concomitant organ pathology. Further perioperative management will often encompass large-scale fluid resuscitation and long-term critical care interventions. This makes a comparison of anesthetic choice and analgesic techniques and their isolated impact on outcomes difficult.

There are, however, a few categories of isolated orthopedic trauma, whereby the literature is more mature concerning perioperative outcomes. In this context, we will present a narrative review on the body of evidence as it relates to anesthesia-related outcomes in patients with hip fractures, rib fractures, and other extremity fractures.

THE CHOICE OF ANESTHESIA TYPE IN TRAUMA PATIENTS

There are general concerns related to the choice of anesthetic technique for orthopedic trauma; these include the patient's overall burden of injury, comorbidities, and the planned procedure, among others.

General anesthesia is commonly *initially* used in severe multi-trauma, especially in patients having emergent surgery on more than one area of the body. Multiple injuries can complicate the feasibility and safety of regional techniques, as well as successful and adequate pain control; Length of surgery can be unpredictable, fluid resuscitation may be massive and the central nervous, as well as the respiratory system, might be affected requiring control of the airway. Similarly, patient positioning for the selected surgical procedures and the need for prolonged tourniquet times or other interventions such as transesophageal echocardiogram to guide fluid management can also necessitate a general anesthetic with endotracheal intubation. Injury burden can also complicate positioning needed for safe block placement or neuraxial anesthesia. Indeed, patient cooperation cannot be assumed, and the risk of aspiration with deep sedation, or diminished safety profile may also require general anesthesia with a secured airway.

Patient-specific physiologic and injury-induced derangements will also often preclude the use of regional anesthetic techniques. Severe hypovolemia, often due to significant preoperative or intraoperative blood loss may lead to patient intolerance of the sympathectomy associated with neuraxial techniques. Existing nerve injuries in trauma patients can be masked by neuraxial or nerve blocks[10] and, the potential for delayed recognition should be discussed with patients and surgeons. Severe trauma may preclude regional anesthesia use until the patient is hemodynamically stabilized.

In many of these patients, pre and postoperative pain control presents additional opportunities for regional techniques, with the goal to improve mobility and reduce the sympathetic response to pain.[11,12] However, concern for the inability to detect a potential compartment syndrome is also frequently being voiced by surgeons when PNBs are involved, but this might not be entirely evidence based.[13]

Coagulopathy is common, whether due to medication, trauma burden, aggressive resuscitation, or medical comorbidities. Many neuraxial and regional techniques are relatively contraindicated in these patients, and this should be taken into consideration. Additionally, plans for postoperative anticoagulation may inform the decision on the safety of regional anesthesia.

HIP FRACTURE

Although hip fractures account for only ~20% of fractures, the high morbidity and need for operative intervention make this entity an area of continuous study. Conservative estimates suggest that approximately 300,000 hip fractures occur in the United States on an annual basis. Population trends predict that the annual number of this injury could total 1,000,000 by the year 2040 in the US alone.[14] Additionally, hip fractures are associated with advanced age and high comorbidity burden, making the perioperative care of these patients, particularly challenging.

Early retrospective reviews[15] suggested that regional anesthesia was associated with lower odds of inpatient mortality and pulmonary complications when compared with general anesthesia. Specifically, an advantage was seen in those with intertrochanteric compared with femoral neck fractures. Later studies by the same group looked at more than 50,000 patients who had received general or regional anesthesia and found no difference in 30-day mortality. Authors did, however, determine a very modest reduction in length of stay (6.2 vs 6.6 days)[16]

When further examining morbidity related to hip fracture Fields[17] and Basques[18] both reported a significant reduction in thromboembolic complications with the utilization of spinal anesthesia over general anesthesia in separate studies with more than 6000 cases. Basques specifically focused on patients greater than 70 years of age. When applied to a population of older hip fracture patients with dementia though, Seitz and colleagues, could not confirm these findings.[19]

More recently, in a systematic review of studies in patients with hip fracture, Guay and colleagues[20] demonstrated that spinal anesthesia decreased the incidence of hypertension, while no difference in postoperative outcomes including mortality, myocardial infarction, congestive heart failure, thromboembolic complications, and length of stay (LOS) was found. These results have previously been called into question due to low quality of evidence, substantial bias, and lack of statistical power. Additionally, a time period of over 3 decades may not accurately reflect current practice.

A retrospective cohort study by Malhas and colleagues[21] in 2019 again examined 90-day mortality following hip fracture surgery and found a weak association toward decreased mortality with spinal anesthesia over general anesthesia. In their study, spinal anesthesia was also associated with decreased morbidity, specifically finding lower rates of major blood loss, pulmonary embolism (PE), and LOS.

The impact of PNBs on outcomes in hip fracture has been summarized by Guay and colleagues using data collected up to 2020. By reviewing ~50 randomized control trials (RCTs) they found that PNB had proven benefit in pain reduction, risk of acute confusional state, risk of chest infection, and time to first mobilization, as well as a small reduction in anesthetic cost.[22] They found no difference in myocardial infarction or mortality, although their analyses for these outcomes were insufficiently powered.

In summary, the lack of overall conclusive signal has driven researchers to pool evidence from multiple RCTs to help provide robust evidence on best anesthesia practices.[1] In 2019, a consensus statement[23] summarized the intermittent research with suggestions to help guide care. Relevant to the current discussion, the authors determined that;

1. when available, regional analgesic techniques (PNBs) before surgery in patients with hip fractures are recommended,
2. large-scale observational data seem to indicate that regional anesthesia is associated with lower 30-day morbidity (including decreased surgical site infection, decreased deep venous thrombosis (DVT), and shorter LOS)
3. regional anesthesia was shown to be associated with lower odds of pulmonary complications and inpatient mortality among patients with hip fracture (likely driven by a trend toward better outcomes in patients with intertrochanteric fractures)
4. large-scale RCTs examining regional to general anesthesia for hip fracture specifically are rare and outcomes studied limited.[24]

Although not specifically in patients with hip *fracture*, the ICAROS guidelines additionally recommended neuraxial over general anesthesia for hip and knee *arthroplasty*, with the strongest recommendation for hip arthroplasty, based on best current evidence.[9,25] While extrapolating this data to hip fractures may be somewhat limited, it should be considered in the overall discussion.

Furthermore, at the time of the publication process, the results of the "Regional versus General Anesthesia for Promoting Independence after Hip Fracture" (REGAIN) trial were published in the New England Journal of Medicine.[26] This large prospective trial aimed to provide adequately powered data to evaluate any difference in long-term outcomes between neuraxial and general anesthesia in patients undergoing hip surgery. Enrolling 1600 patients, the authors showed no difference between the 2 groups in terms of the primary outcomes (mortality and recovery of ambulation at 60 days) supporting the ability of the anesthesia provider to choose the anesthetic technique best suited to their patients' wishes and case details. Limitations, however, included: a relatively healthy patient population (leading to a smaller than expected incidence in the primary outcomes, thus reducing power), a large percentage (13%) of study participants who received general instead of the assigned regional technique, and the overall heterogeneity of anesthetic regimens allowed within both groups. Importantly, the study was not powered sufficiently to detect differences in complications, which might be argued is a more mechanistically appropriate outcome to study. Neuraxial anesthesia for example, is associated with sympathectomy-induced blood pressure control and thus reduced blood loss and tissue perfusion, decreases in inflammatory mediators, and improved pulmonary mechanics due to avoidance of intubation. Indeed, some of the data in the REGAIN study suggest that there are higher rates of some complications in the general group such as those affecting the pulmonary and renal systems. In addition, a growing body of evidence indicates the benefits of regional anesthesia for the prevention of numerous complications significant to the patients' perioperative health and resource utilization.[9] In contrast, the outcomes of mortality and the ability to walk after 60 days, although important, are mechanistically difficult to explain by the choice of anesthetic as there are numerous, and more targeted interventions (ie, intensive monitoring and rehabilitation) used to affect these outcomes after surgery.

RIB FRACTURE

Rib fractures are common in orthopedic trauma and represent a substantial health burden, affecting nearly 1 in 5 trauma patients. While chest injury contributes to approximately 25% of deaths in trauma patients, mortality has been found to be directly correlated with the number of ribs fractured. These injuries often lead to long-term consequences and therefore have been the topic of numerous investigations.[27]

Patients with a large trauma burden will often have multiple procedures, but only a fraction will require surgical interventions for rib fractures, per se. Rib plating is often reserved for flail chest and displaced fractures,[28] and will routinely involve a general anesthetic. The role of regional anesthesia in these patients therefore focuses on analgesia that will provide long-term pain relief, and importantly, prevent excessive splinting and its sequelae, including pneumonia and atelectasis. Multiple regional anesthetic options have been proposed, including neuraxial (epidural)-based techniques and PNBs.

The most robust area of anesthesia research in rib fracture outcomes investigates how regional anesthesia affects outcomes and systemic pain relief, and further explores the superiority of specific regional analgesic techniques. Traditionally, epidural analgesia has been the regional anesthetic technique with the best evidence of efficacy in rib fractures. Catheter-based techniques have demonstrated superior pain relief when compared with systemic opioids, and importantly, a lower incidence of pulmonary-related complications. This has not translated into an observable effect on mortality. With the advent of increased interest in ultrasound-guided techniques, clinicians have started to compare epidural approaches with several PNBs. These commonly include intercostal nerve blocks, paravertebral nerve blocks, erector spinae plane (ESP) blocks, and serratus anterior plane blocks. PNBs may be preferable in the trauma population as thoracic epidural may not be appropriate in the setting of common conditions such as coagulopathy, sepsis, hypovolemia/hypotension, and head injuries. Peripheral techniques offer an attractive option for these patients.

Using a large database in 2017, Malekpour suggested that epidural anesthesia and paravertebral nerve blocks did not produce significant differences in outcomes, and even showed an association between the use of a paravertebral block and improved outcomes.[29] However, the authors did admit that these results could be biased due to the selection of healthier patients for PNB. A further meta-analysis performed in 2019 showed that thoracic epidurals provided superior analgesia compared with paravertebral and intercostal blocks, as well as systemic IV pain medications.[30] No differences were observed for secondary endpoints such as length of ICU stay, length of mechanical ventilation, or pulmonary complications. Again, the quality of this study was questioned, and precluded the drafting of a firm recommendation.[30] ESP blocks are similarly lacking solid evidence, likely due to their novelty. However, it has been suggested that they are highly efficacious techniques for rib fracutres.[31] Serratus anterior plane blocks may also be beneficial in anterior rib fractures.

While the mentioned PNBs provide good initial relief, they suffer from a limited duration of action and the need to repeat the procedure if no catheter is used. Liposomal bupivacaine, first FDA-approved in 2011 has been studied with great interest for its suitability to provide long-term pain relief without the need for continuous catheter placement. Despite significant concern that the liposomal formulation might not be superior to plain bupivacaine in many settings,[32] Sheets and colleagues explored its use compared with epidural analgesia and found that patients who received intercostal nerve blocks with liposomal bupivacaine required intubation less frequently and had shorter ICU and hospital status compared with patients who received epidural analgesia.[33] While their results indicated that liposomal bupivacaine might be equal or superior to epidural analgesia, they did not compare liposomal bupivacaine to its plain version, and thus no firm conclusions to its role can be drawn.

Concern surrounding spinal neurologic injury and cardiovascular consequences potentially associated with thoracic epidural analgesia has nevertheless continued to raise interest in PNBs and led to a decrease in epidural use for rib fractures in the recent past. Fewer, and less serious complications seen with PNBs as compared with epidurals continue to make their use enticing, even more so when considering the widespread use of anticoagulation in the elderly population. These blocks are increasingly being used despite a lack of evidence base.[30] Therefore, the current state of solid evidence surrounding outcomes in rib fracture may be best described as it was by El-Boghdadly: "too many options, too little evidence."[34]

OTHER EXTREMITY FRACTURE

Isolated upper and lower extremity fractures are often amenable to regional anesthesia. While avoiding a general anesthetic with regional anesthesia is often complicated by polytrauma and surgical needs, regional anesthesia is well accepted and validated in providing superior analgesia for intraoperative as well as pre- and post-surgical pain.

Clavicle fractures

Historically, fractures of the proximal and mid clavicle often necessitated general anesthesia, while distal clavicle and shoulder interventions were often performed under regional anesthesia. Due to the innervation of the clavicle, sparing is often seen with interscalene blocks (that do not include the supraclavicular branches of the superficial cervical plexus) along the more proximal clavicle. Repeated studies have now investigated a single-shot technique of superficial cervical plexus and interscalene block that allowed patients to tolerate regional anesthesia for all clavicle procedures.[35] The combined block seems to be a reasonable alternative to general anesthesia with an interscalene brachial plexus block, and superficial cervical plexus blockade alone provides good postoperative analgesia when used in patients receiving general anesthesia. However, in deciding whether regional anesthesia is used as the primary anesthetic for this surgery, the anesthesiologist must consider the proximity of the surgery to the airway, assess the need and ease for airway manipulation during surgery, and take into account the clinical implications of phrenic paralysis that almost invariably accompanies interscalene blockade.

Upper extremity fractures

Most procedures for upper extremity fractures can be easily performed under brachial plexus blocks, with additional intercostobrachial blockade for upper arm surgery or tourniquet pain. For shorter procedures, a tourniquet is well tolerated without the addition of an intercostobrachial block (for tourniquet times less than 60 to 75 minutes). While numerous approaches to brachial plexus blocks have been described, supraclavicular, infraclavicular, and axillary blocks all provide reliable analgesia. Axillary blocks have been shown to offer superior analgesia and satisfactory anesthesia for upper limb trauma surgery when compared with general anesthesia.[36] Closed reduction of phalanx fractures can often be performed with a digital block.

While single-shot PNBs are well studied for intraoperative and immediate postoperative pain, continuous catheter-based techniques continue to be an area of active research. For upper arm surgery, the interscalene block has been shown to be superior to opioid-based analgesia, but was itself found to be inferior to continuous catheter-based blocks in moderately and extremely painful surgeries.[37] Particular benefit may be seen with upper extremity reimplantation surgery, as the sympathectomy associated with the block may improve blood flow across vascular anastomoses. Similarly, the use of continuous infraclavicular perineural blocks is well validated for elbow surgery. For surgical procedures distal to the elbow, brachial plexus catheter infusions have been shown to provide less impressive analgesia. Evidence is still lacking on the possible benefit of other brachial plexus blocks in these situations.[37]

Lower extremity fractures

Lower extremity surgery will often necessitate blockade of multiple nerves innervating the dermatomes and osteotomes of the legs, but can reliably provide surgical conditions with minimal patient repositioning. Injuries can range from distal tibia, fibula, and foot fractures to proximal femur fractures. Femur fractures can carry a mortality as high as 25% and can be accompanied by massive blood loss. Again, patient injury burden will often dictate the choice of general versus regional anesthesia, but nonetheless repeated RCTs have shown excellent and superior pain control postoperatively when regional techniques are used. In isolated fractures, regional techniques have been found to be a viable option instead of general anesthesia.

Egol and colleagues found higher patient functional scores, and lower acute and chronic pain in patients followed for 1 year after distal radial fracture repair under regional anesthesia compared with general approaches.[38] Satisfaction and postoperative pain management have been shown to be improved for lower extremity fractures in the first 24 hours in patients who received PNBs as part of their analgesic regimen, compared with systemic analgesia.[38,39]

Nonetheless, utilization of PNBs in lower extremity trauma surgery remains low, estimated at ~10% by Brovman and colleagues, with the majority being neuraxial anesthetics.[13] The same group also found no significant differences in 30-day mortality and postoperative complications for regional versus general anesthesia for patients with lower extremity orthopedic fractures.

While prolonged motor blockade is seen as an unwanted side effect in outpatient procedures, whereby expedited return to mobility is the goal, many orthopedic trauma patients will have longer recovery periods and benefit from prolonged analgesia. Continuous PNBs, especially in proximal lower extremity injuries, can be problematic due to the need for multiple catheters to block the transmission of numerous nerves innervating the leg.[37] For foot and ankle surgery, the use of continuous PNBs has clearly demonstrated superiority to other analgesic regimens, including single-shot nerve blocks. It has been shown to decrease hospital costs and LOS. Additionally, several studies have shown that regional anesthesia for foot surgery is safe and leads to reduced perioperative opioid requirements.[40]

In general, the summary of good quality evidence seems to be that in the great majority of blocks reviewed for lower extremity surgery, results show reduced opioid consumption and pain scores as well as increased patient satisfaction.[37] For specific surgical procedures, PNBs can also be used to avoid general anesthesia. Complications are rare.[40] The widespread utility for continuous catheter techniques continues to be explored and likely precludes recommendation at this time.

SUMMARY

Anesthesia for the management of orthopedic trauma continues to be a dynamic field that is quickly evolving as new techniques become available. The literature is starting to mature in specific fields such as hip[15,17,18,20,21,23,24,41,42] and patients with rib fracture,[28,29,31,33,34] whereby regional anesthetic and analgesic techniques may provide benefits. Additionally, some benefits regarding lower morbidity, especially cardiac complications, pulmonary complications, thromboembolic phenomenon, bleeding, and critical care admissions have been observed.[43]

Despite remaining questions precluding robust recommendation in favor of regional techniques, inferiority of regional anesthesia and analgesia over their alternatives has not been shown. As previously stated, "one would be hard-pressed to conclude that outcomes are worse with regional techniques compared with alternative approaches, that is, general anesthesia or systemic analgesia."[43] While the literature on the impact on outcomes of these interventions remains far from definitive, they have almost all proven to be viable options for effective use in the correct patient population.

Today, it seems short- and long-term benefits are often overlooked in lieu of less effective opioid-based regimens to avoid uncommon complications and slowed workflow. A familiarity with new techniques and experience with their execution and workflow will help to further advance the specialty.

Regional anesthesia-related complications

Compartment syndrome is a feared condition in trauma patients that can evolve into a true surgical emergency. Historically, there has been concern surrounding the possibility of delayed diagnosis with the use of regional anesthesia, as the patient would be unable to alert the provider to intensifying pain which has been described as a hallmark of the syndrome. This topic is covered in detail in the *Acute Extremity Compartment Syndrome and (Regional) Anesthesia – the monster under the bed* chapter of this special issue.

Block-related nerve injuries are very rare (0.4 per 1000 blocks)[44] and mostly transient and subclinical. In fact, most nerve injuries observed may not be related to PNB[45] but can also be linked to surgical and patient-related factors.[5,44,46–51] While acknowledging nerve injury as a potential complication, current evidence suggests that regional anesthesia provides efficient anesthesia and analgesia for many procedures, while indications and applications are rising, as are advanced in training and practice techniques.[5]

REGIONAL ANESTHESIA LIMITATIONS/CONTRAINDICATIONS

Contraindications to regional anesthesia in *trauma* include standard contraindications to regional anesthesia (patient refusal, allergy to local anesthetic, infection in the area) but also should be cognizant of increased safety concerns in a trauma setting.

In these patients contraindications should include the following[10]:

- Patient is heavily sedated or obtunded* or when consent cannot reliably be obtained.
- Safety concerns due to uncooperative patients
- Interference with ATLS resuscitation
- Inability to position the patient for the procedure
- Polytrauma patient whereby systemic approach is more practical
- Injuries mandating general anesthesia for definitive surgical treatment
- Lack of appropriate training and equipment

*While called into question with the continuous improvement of ultrasound-guided techniques, the American Society of Regional Anesthesia (ASRA) still recommends against performing blocks in anesthetized or heavily sedated patients, unless benefits plainly outweigh risks.[10]

FUTURE AREAS OF STUDY

Ultimately, and despite many advanced in the field, utilization rates of regional anesthesia remain fairly low.[52] However, the benefits of regional techniques have been recognized by non-anesthesiologists and are for example, deployed in emergency rooms across the country.[53] The requirement of physician training and skill for successful PNB utilization may be a possible driver of low utilization. Given the continuing progress in anesthesia practice, including both regional and general anesthesia techniques, the incidence of severe postoperative complications attributable to anesthesia has become relatively rare. This presents a challenge for scientific research, as large sample sizes are needed to detect any potential differences in outcome. In particular, when addressing harm, it is well established that evidence from randomized trials (RCTs) alone is often imprecise, indirect, or inapplicable, requiring nonrandomized studies of interventions to complement RCTs when informing clinical decision making.[54,55]

Future trials should also focus on modern clinical settings, including the implementation of fast-track pathways in the context of improving the quality of care. Such clinical pathways often rely on the implementation of regional anesthesia techniques, anticipating best practice in pain management and rapid postoperative recovery.[56] Many of these trials are underway, and results are eagerly awaited.

DISCLOSURE

S. G. Memtsoudis is a one-time consultant for Sandoz Inc. and the holder US Patent Multicatheter Infusion System. US-2017 to 0,361,063. He is the owner of SGM Consulting, LLC and Centauros Healthcare Analytics and Consulting. S. G. Memtsoudis is also a shareholder in Parvizi Surgical Innovations LLC and HATH. None of the above relations influenced the conduct of the present project. P. Gerner and C. Cozowicz have no conflicts of interest to disclose.

CLINICS CARE POINTS

- When possible, using regional anesthesia techniques before surgery in patients with hip fracture is recommended.
- Regional anesthesia for hip fracture, rib fracture, and isolated extremity fracture has shown outcome benefits.
- The decision to use regional anesthesia in trauma surgery patients must take into consideration surgical and patient factors.
- Block-related nerve injury is extremely rare when performed by experienced practitioners.

REFERENCES

1. Cozowicz C, Poeran J, Memtsoudis SG. Epidemiology, trends, and disparities in regional anaesthesia for orthopaedic surgery. Br J Anaesth 2015;115(Suppl 2): ii57–67.
2. Rodgers A, Walker N, Schug S, et al. Reduction of postoperative mortality and morbidity with epidural or spinal anaesthesia: results from overview of randomised trials. BMJ 2000;321(7275):1493.
3. Kehlet H. The modifying effect of anesthetic technique on the metabolic and endocrine responses to anesthesia and surgery. Acta Anaesthesiol Belg 1988; 39(3):143–6.

4. Kehlet H. Modification of responses to surgery by neural blockade. Neural blockade. Philadelphia: Lippincott-Raven; 1998. p. 129–75.

5. Brull R, McCartney CJ, Chan VW, et al. Neurological complications after regional anesthesia: contemporary estimates of risk. Anesth Analg 2007;104(4):965–74.

6. Cook TM, Counsell D, Wildsmith JA, et al. Major complications of central neuraxial block: report on the Third National Audit Project of the Royal College of Anaesthetists. Br J Anaesth 2009;102(2):179–90.

7. Holte K, Kehlet H. Epidural anaesthesia and analgesia - effects on surgical stress responses and implications for postoperative nutrition. Clin Nutr 2002;21(3):199–206.

8. Barreveld A, Witte J, Chahal H, et al. Preventive analgesia by local anesthetics: the reduction of postoperative pain by peripheral nerve blocks and intravenous drugs. Anesth Analg 2013;116(5):1141–61.

9. Memtsoudis SG, Cozowicz C, Bekeris J, et al. Peripheral nerve block anesthesia/analgesia for patients undergoing primary hip and knee arthroplasty: recommendations from the International Consensus on Anesthesia-Related Outcomes after Surgery (ICAROS) group based on a systematic review and meta-analysis of current literature. Reg Anesth Pain Med 2021. https://doi.org/10.1136/rapm-2021-102750.

10. Fleming I, Egeler C. Regional Anesthesia For Trauma: An Update. Continuing Education Anaesth Crit Care Pain 2014;14(3):136–41.

11. O'Neill J, Helwig E. Postoperative Management of the Physiological Effects of Spinal Anesthesia. J Perianesth Nurs 2016;31(4):330–9.

12. Zhu L, Tian C, Li M, et al. The stress response and anesthetic potency of unilateral spinal anesthesia for total Hip Replacement in geriatric patients. Pakistan J Pharm Sci 2014;27(6 Suppl):2029–34.

13. Brovman EY, Wallace FC, Weaver MJ, et al. Anesthesia Type Is Not Associated With Postoperative Complications in the Care of Patients With Lower Extremity Traumatic Fractures. Anesth Analg 2019;129(4):1034–42.

14. Melton LJ. Hip fractures: a worldwide problem today and tomorrow. Bone 1993;14(Suppl 1):S1–8.

15. Neuman MD, Silber JH, Elkassabany NM, et al. Comparative effectiveness of regional versus general anesthesia for hip fracture surgery in adults. Anesthesiology 2012;117(1):72–92.

16. Neuman MD, Rosenbaum PR, Ludwig JM, et al. Anesthesia technique, mortality, and length of stay after hip fracture surgery. JAMA 2014;311(24):2508–17.

17. Fields AC, Dieterich JD, Buterbaugh K, et al. Short-term complications in hip fracture surgery using spinal versus general anaesthesia. Injury 2015;46(4):719–23.

18. Basques BA, Bohl DD, Golinvaux NS, et al. General versus spinal anaesthesia for patients aged 70 years and older with a fracture of the hip. bone Jt J 2015;97-b(5):689–95.

19. Seitz DP, Gill SS, Bell CM, et al. Postoperative medical complications associated with anesthesia in older adults with dementia. J Am Geriatr Soc 2014;62(11):2102–9.

20. Guay J, Parker MJ, Gajendragadkar PR, et al. Anaesthesia for hip fracture surgery in adults. Cochrane Database Syst Rev 2016;2:Cd000521. https://doi.org/10.1002/14651858.CD000521.pub3.

21. Malhas L, Perlas A, Tierney S, et al. The effect of anesthetic technique on mortality and major morbidity after hip fracture surgery: a retrospective, propensity-score matched-pairs cohort study. Reg Anesth Pain Med 2019;44(9):847–53.

22. Guay J, Kopp S. Peripheral nerve blocks for hip fractures in adults. Cochrane Database Syst Rev 2020;11(11):Cd001159.

23. Soffin EM, Gibbons MM, Wick EC, et al. Evidence Review Conducted for the Agency for Healthcare Research and Quality Safety Program for Improving Surgical Care and Recovery: Focus on Anesthesiology for Hip Fracture Surgery. Anesth Analg 2019;128(6):1107–17.
24. Neuman MD, Ellenberg SS, Sieber FE, et al. Regional versus General Anesthesia for Promoting Independence after Hip Fracture (REGAIN): protocol for a pragmatic, international multicentre trial. BMJ Open 2016;6(11):e013473. https://doi.org/10.1136/bmjopen-2016-013473.
25. Memtsoudis SG, Cozowicz C, Bekeris J, et al. Anaesthetic care of patients undergoing primary hip and knee arthroplasty: consensus recommendations from the International Consensus on Anaesthesia-Related Outcomes after Surgery group (ICAROS) based on a systematic review and meta-analysis. Br J Anaesth 2019; 123(3):269–87.
26. Neuman MD, Feng R, Carson JL, et al. Spinal Anesthesia or General Anesthesia for Hip Surgery in Older Adults. N Engl J Med 2021;385(22):2025–35.
27. Williams A, Bigham C, Marchbank A. Anaesthetic and surgical management of rib fractures. BJA Educ 2020;20(10):332–40.
28. Kasotakis G, Hasenboehler EA, Streib EW, et al. Operative fixation of rib fractures after blunt trauma: A practice management guideline from the Eastern Association for the Surgery of Trauma. J Trauma Acute Care Surg 2017;82(3):618–26.
29. Malekpour M, Hashmi A, Dove J, et al. Analgesic Choice in Management of Rib Fractures: Paravertebral Block or Epidural Analgesia? Anesth Analg 2017;124(6): 1906–11.
30. Peek J, DPJ Smeeing, Hietbrink F, et al. Comparison of analgesic interventions for traumatic rib fractures: a systematic review and meta-analysis. Eur J Trauma Emerg Surg 2019;45(4):597–622.
31. Adhikary SD, Liu WM, Fuller E, et al. The effect of erector spinae plane block on respiratory and analgesic outcomes in multiple rib fractures: a retrospective cohort study. Anaesthesia 2019;74(5):585–93.
32. Hussain N, Brull R, Sheehy B, et al. Perineural Liposomal Bupivacaine Is Not Superior to Nonliposomal Bupivacaine for Peripheral Nerve Block Analgesia. Anesthesiology 2021;134(2):147–64.
33. Sheets NW, Davis JW, Dirks RC, et al. Intercostal Nerve Block with Liposomal Bupivacaine vs Epidural Analgesia for the Treatment of Traumatic Rib Fracture. J Am Coll Surg 2020;231(1):150–4.
34. El-Boghdadly K, Wiles MD. Regional anaesthesia for rib fractures: too many choices, too little evidence. Anaesthesia 2019;74(5):564–8.
35. Ryan DJ, Iofin N, Furgiuele D, et al. Regional anesthesia for clavicle fracture surgery is safe and effective. J Shoulder Elbow Surg 2021;30(7):e356–60.
36. O'Donnell BD, Ryan H, O'Sullivan O, et al. Ultrasound-guided axillary brachial plexus block with 20 milliliters local anesthetic mixture versus general anesthesia for upper limb trauma surgery: an observer-blinded, prospective, randomized, controlled trial. Anesth Analg 2009;109(1):279–83.
37. Aguirre J, Del Moral A, Cobo I, et al. The role of continuous peripheral nerve blocks. Anesthesiol Res Pract 2012;2012:560879.
38. Egol KA, Soojian MG, Walsh M, et al. Regional anesthesia improves outcome after distal radius fracture fixation over general anesthesia. J Orthop Trauma 2012; 26(9):545–9.
39. Elkassabany N, Cai LF, Mehta S, et al. Does Regional Anesthesia Improve the Quality of Postoperative Pain Management and the Quality of Recovery in

Patients Undergoing Operative Repair of Tibia and Ankle Fractures? J Orthop Trauma 2015;29(9):404–9.

40. Bugada D, Ghisi D, Mariano ER. Continuous regional anesthesia: a review of perioperative outcome benefits. Minerva Anestesiol 2017;83(10):1089–100.

41. Guay J, Kopp S. Peripheral nerve blocks for hip fractures in adults. Cochrane Database Syst Rev 2020;11:CD001159.

42. Tung YC, Hsu YH, Chang GM. The Effect of Anesthetic Type on Outcomes of Hip Fracture Surgery: A Nationwide Population-Based Study. Medicine (Baltimore) 2016;95(14):e3296.

43. Memtsoudis SG, Liu SS. Do neuraxial techniques affect perioperative outcomes? The story of vantage points and number games. Anesth Analg 2014;119(3): 501–2.

44. Barrington MJ, Watts SA, Gledhill SR, et al. Preliminary results of the Australasian Regional Anaesthesia Collaboration: a prospective audit of more than 7000 peripheral nerve and plexus blocks for neurologic and other complications. Reg Anesth Pain Med 2009;34(6):534–41, 534-541.

45. Yajnik M, Kou A, Mudumbai SC, et al. Peripheral nerve blocks are not associated with increased risk of perioperative peripheral nerve injury in a Veterans Affairs inpatient surgical population. Reg Anesth Pain Med 2019;44(1):81–5.

46. Jeng C, Torrillo T, Rosenblatt M. Complications of peripheral nerve blocks. Br J Anaesth 2010;105(suppl_1):i97–107.

47. Barrington MJ, Snyder GL. Neurologic complications of regional anesthesia. Curr Opin Anesthesiology 2011;24(5):554–60.

48. Neal JM, Barrington MJ, Brull R, et al. The Second ASRA Practice Advisory on Neurologic Complications Associated With Regional Anesthesia and Pain Medicine: Executive Summary 2015. Reg Anesth Pain Med 2015;40(5):401–30.

49. Walker KJ, McGrattan K, Aas-Eng K, et al. Ultrasound guidance for peripheral nerve blockade. Cochrane Database Syst Rev 2009;4.

50. Fredrickson MJ, Kilfoyle DH. Neurological complication analysis of 1000 ultrasound guided peripheral nerve blocks for elective orthopaedic surgery: a prospective study. Anaesthesia 2009;64(8):836–44.

51. Sites BD, Taenzer AH, Herrick MD, et al. Incidence of local anesthetic systemic toxicity and postoperative neurologic symptoms associated with 12,668 ultrasound-guided nerve blocks: an analysis from a prospective clinical registry. 2012.

52. Cozowicz C, Poeran J, Zubizarreta N, et al. Trends in the Use of Regional Anesthesia: Neuraxial and Peripheral Nerve Blocks. Reg Anesth Pain Med 2016; 41(1):43–9.

53. Kolodychuk N, Krebs JC, Stenberg R, et al. Fascia Iliaca Blocks Performed in the Emergency Department Decrease Opioid Consumption and Length of Stay in Hip Fracture Patients. J Orthop Trauma 2021. https://doi.org/10.1097/BOT. 0000000000002220.

54. O'Neil M, Berkman N, Hartling L, et al. Observational evidence and strength of evidence domains: case examples. Syst Rev 2014;3:35. https://doi.org/10. 1186/2046-4053-3-35.

55. Chou R, Aronson N, Atkins D, et al. AHRQ series paper 4: assessing harms when comparing medical interventions: AHRQ and the effective health-care program. J Clin Epidemiol 2010;63(5):502–12.

56. Mancel L, Van Loon K, Lopez AM. Role of regional anesthesia in Enhanced Recovery After Surgery (ERAS) protocols. Curr Opin Anaesthesiol 2021;34(5): 616–25.

Rebound Pain After Peripheral Nerve Blockade— Bad Timing or Rude Awakening?

Alexander Stone, MD[a,b], Philipp Lirk, MD, PhD[a,*],
Kamen Vlassakov, MD[a]

KEYWORDS

- Nerve block • Rebound pain • Nerve injury

KEY POINTS

- Patients often experience moderate to severe pain after peripheral nerve block resolution.
- This seems more common after bone surgery, in patients who are younger, female, and in whom a dense block wears off during a time period when nociceptive stimuli are still intense, and postsurgical pain is normally expected to be moderate to severe.
- Management is largely by anticipation, modification of block duration, implementation of multimodal analgesic regimens, and patient education.
- Even though there is limited translational evidence for a separate pathophysiologic process potentially involving proinflammatory and neurotoxic effects of local anesthetics, the clinical relevance of these respective contributions is unclear and probably minor.
- To the best of our knowledge today, the main factors in the occurrence of rebound pain are a nerve block resolution that is timed suboptimally and a poorly planned transition to the subsequent pain therapy regimen.

INTRODUCTION

Rebound pain or pain after regional anesthesia/analgesia resolution is a phenomenon that is attracting greater attention, especially with the increasingly ambitious goals of health care providers and institutions to enhance recovery, spare opioids, and reduce hospital length of stay after major surgery. Definitions vary widely and go beyond the semantics, whereby "rebound" may not be the most accurate descriptor (consider "recurrent"), or the timeline, which may span from 12 to more than 24 hours postoperatively (why not 48 hours?), but is most often implicitly defined as "when the block

Conflicts of interest: None.
[a] Department of Anesthesiology, Perioperative and Pain Medicine, Brigham and Women's Hospital, Harvard Medical School, 75 Francis Street, Boston, MA 02115, USA; [b] Department of Anesthesiology, Hospital for Special Surgery, 535 East 70th Street, New York, NY 10021, USA
* Corresponding author. Department of Anesthesiology, Perioperative and Pain Medicine, Brigham and Women's Hospital, Harvard Medical School, 75 Francis Street, Boston, MA 02115.
E-mail address: plirk@bwh.harvard.edu

Anesthesiology Clin 40 (2022) 445–454
https://doi.org/10.1016/j.anclin.2022.03.002
1932-2275/22/© 2022 Elsevier Inc. All rights reserved.
anesthesiology.theclinics.com

wears off." A more important question would be if rebound pain is a phenomenon with distinct pathophysiology or simply predictable surgical pain unveiled by premature resolution of nerve conduction blockade. The published literature offers a variety of qualifications and suggested mechanisms ranging from regional anesthesia "side effect" to neuroinflammation caused by a nerve block. But in the absence of any known specific pathologic findings associated with rebound pain, why would we not interpret it in the most obvious way—as the result of a nerve block with a duration shorter than that of the intense and expected postsurgical nociceptive stimuli? Just like the dreaded situation of a spinal anesthetic wearing off before surgery is completed, such a point of view would escalate the status of rebound pain from a side effect to a complication attributable to inadequate postsurgical analgesia planning.

But how do we prepare sufficiently well for the need for intense postoperative analgesia when pain trajectories remain somewhat unpredictable and critically dependent on a complex interplay of individual psychosocial and physiologic factors?

DEFINITION

There is a range of definitions for rebound pain which varies in specificity and ability to be measured. Yet, there are some common themes in the proposed definitions of rebound pain.[1] Timing is a critical factor when considering rebound pain. Most of the definitions state that rebound pain occurs after a previously effective nerve block has resolved.[2–8] Some suggest a discrete time period for rebound pain to occur following block resolution[2,9] with a focus on the first hours after the resolution of the nerve block. Rebound pain is also loosely described as having a fast onset and reaching peak intensity quickly.[6] Many definitions of rebound pain quantify the pain as severe.[1,10] It is generally expected for rebound pain to be transient, though this is not included in most definitions of rebound pain.[11] While some definitions imply that rebound pain is similar in pathophysiology to hyperalgesia,[9] there is little evidence to support that claim, as some degree of hyperalgesia may be a predictable component of postoperative pain.

Operationally, groups have sought to describe and measure rebound pain in various ways. It is important to remember that there is no gold standard for quantifying or even qualitatively measuring rebound pain. William and colleagues used the highest pain score within the first 12 hours of the patient reporting that their nerve block was no longer providing relief, minus the pain score the patient reported the last time when their nerve block was providing relief.[2] Galos and colleagues collected pain scores at 2-hour intervals and compared the group of patients who received a nerve block to patients who did not.[4] Barry and colleagues reported an incidence of rebound pain in their patient cohort and used a definition of patients who experienced severe pain (self-reported pain score >6 out of 10) at home after the last pain score in the postanesthesia care unit (PACU) before discharge was reported as mild.[6] More recently, Woo and colleagues quantified rebound pain by the lowest pain score before block resolution subtracted from the highest pain score during the first 12 hours after block resolution.[8]

The various operational definitions present significant limitations. They rely on patient-reported pain score at specific points in time and are often retrospective. Another limitation is that they do not account selectively for pain at rest versus pain with activity. Physical therapy is more likely to start between 12 and 24 hours after surgery and can influence pain scores. This also typically coincides with the block resolution for a good reason—recovery of motor function and proprioception—posing the question if rebound pain would be significantly different (or present) if/when blocks are anatomically and pharmacologically designed to cause less or no motor block. Additionally, with the exception of the article presented by Williams and colleagues,[2] these definitions do not provide clear criteria for peripheral block resolution, which is highly variable and often not a single point in time. Also, multiple groups have used the peak pain scores during a large time interval following block resolution,[2,6] and have not made attempts to quantify the duration of pain following block resolution.

A criterion often quoted in discussions on rebound pain is that the [increase in] pain has to be clinically significant.[1] However, "clinically significant" can be vague and open to interpretation. The most basic argument would be that rebound pain is clinically significant when rated as severe by the patient.[6,9] Definitions based on peak pain intensity alone are used to support the argument that rebound pain is very prevalent. However, though reported pain intensity can often peak to severe, rebound pain is not typically sustained, as it does neither affect dramatically patient satisfaction and willingness to have nerve blocks in the future, nor the overall satisfaction with the quality of their recovery.[11,12] Pain severe enough to warrant unplanned emergency room visits within 7 days of surgery is rare (occurring in <1% of cases) and is similar between patients who receive peripheral nerve blocks and those who do not.[13]

TRANSLATIONAL EVIDENCE

Preclinical evidence for a distinct pathophysiological mechanism is almost a decade old. Kolarczyk and Williams investigated behavioral changes after a single-shot ropivacaine sciatic nerve block in rats and found transient and modest heat hyperalgesia after block resolution, while tactile withdrawal threshold measured using von Frey hairs, or withdrawal threshold measured using Randall–Selitto testing remained normal. The hyperalgesia was short-lived and only apparent at one timepoint after block resolution (approximately 2–3 seconds decreased thermal withdrawal latency).[3] In a follow-up study, Janda and colleagues performed a secondary subanalysis of 2 preceding animal experiments in rats, and found transient heat hyperalgesia approximately 2 hours after block resolution, which the authors described as "...*transient and clinically insignificant.*"[14] Another piece of evidence was contributed by An and colleagues, who tested bupivacaine with or without dexamethasone for sciatic nerve block in mice, and found that plain bupivacaine was associated with a delayed heat hyperalgesia (1–2 sec decreased thermal withdrawal latency) which became discernible approximately 3 hours after the block had worn off, and was still detectable at 24 hours, after which all values returned to baseline.[15] Of note, An and colleagues performed histopathologic analysis, and found mild axon degeneration in the plain bupivacaine, but not the bupivacaine-plus-dexamethasone group.[15] This is somehow at odds with the potential for neurotoxicity of high-dose dexamethasone proposed by Williams and colleagues.[16]

In conclusion, the effects found in animal experiments are small to moderate in size, but could help explain the transient phenomenon of hyperalgesia following the resolution of a nerve block. These experiments are very important as they single out just the nerve block itself, without confounding surgical pain sources or analgesic administration.

CLINICAL EVIDENCE

Clinical evidence about rebound pain is harder to analyze, because of the reasons mentioned in the preceding paragraphs—nerve blocks are typically administered perioperatively, and patients are concomitantly receiving pain medicines. The nociceptive input due to preexisting pathology and the surgical intervention with the associated tissue injury and inflammation persists in the postoperative period, and will result in pain when uncovered by the nerve block resolution, similar to the conceptual framework of preemptive and preventive analgesia.[17] Rebound pain was brought to center stage by Williams and colleagues, who investigated excessive pain on the resolution of a perioperative femoral nerve block.[2] Interestingly, the longer nerve blocks lasted, the lower the likelihood of developing excessive pain on its resolution.[2] This was later confirmed by Goldstein and colleagues in the setting of single-shot nerve blocks for ankle surgery. Here, the hyperalgesia occurred about 24 hours after the resolution of a block combining bupivacaine and epinephrine.[18] Of note, the pain score after block resolution was, on average, more than 60 mm on the 100 mm visual analog scale (VAS), nearly as high as the peak pain intensity after surgery experienced by the patients who had only received systemic analgesia.[18] Sort and coworkers quantified the pain trajectory of patients following ankle fracture surgery, and found that nerve blocks provided adequate analgesia for anywhere between 8 and 14 hours, followed by a rise in pain levels, up to a numerical rating scale (NRS 0–10) score of 8 to 10 in some patients.[11] These troubling pain scores may represent a genuine pathophysiological process (including both processes in the nerve, as well as other sequelae of surgery, such as increased tissue edema and pressure), or simply inadequate pain therapy. In the latter scenario, the patient recovering from ankle surgery with an effective nerve block is completely pain-free in PACU and is swiftly discharged to the floor or even home. When the nerve block wears off sometime during the first postoperative evening or night, these patients find themselves in a setting poorly equipped to provide efficient and safe titration of strong pain medicine, so such episodes of escalating acute pain end up being treated inadequately. One way to mitigate such situations in inpatient or extended recovery settings would be to mandate evening and morning follow-up visits to all patients who receive single-shot nerve blocks, conducted by a specialized team such as the Acute Postoperative Pain Service. These visits focus on optimizing both scheduled and as needed multimodal analgesia medications, providing smoother transition from lack of sensation to tolerable pain levels, as well as on educating patients and care team, including nurses, physical therapists, and surgeons about expectations and management strategies. Such an approach to collaborative interdisciplinary postoperative pain management was highlighted by Saminiemi and coworkers, who reported on the successful postoperative pain management of patients with open reduction and internal fixation of ankle fractures, whereby both during the hospital stay, and at all timepoints postoperatively, patients had lower pain scores and lower narcotic consumption.[19] In a mixed cohort of orthopedic surgeries performed under regional anesthesia, between 40% and 50% of patients reported moderate to severe pain once the block wore off,[20] but there was no description of the postoperative pain management protocol. These tasks prove more challenging when the patients are discharged home early after surgery with working neural blockade. The full scope of block resolution is hard to explain and often remains incompletely understood. Paramount is to give patients well-constructed written instructions, as well as provide access to pain medications and expert providers if in need. Educating patient expectations will be discussed later in discussion, but providing a simplified algorithm for timely, effective, and safe self-treatment with multimodal analgesics is critical. Moreover, modern communication platforms extend the opportunity to substitute the inpatient visits described above with virtual ones. However, it is also clear that the virtual and in-person visits described here present logistical and staffing challenges and may remain beyond the present means of many practices. Additionally, more evidence is needed that such approaches will be effective in managing rebound pain, enhancing further functional recovery, and improving patient satisfaction.

Another clinical approach to mitigating or even eliminating the rebound pain phenomenon would be to prolong nerve block effects beyond the point of significant nociceptive input from the surgical or pathologic injury site(s). Many different strategies have been applied, including adjuvants and continuous nerve blocks. While continuous nerve blocks are widely adopted and seem to be most versatile and intuitively superior, the reality is that they are also most expertise-, labor- and material-intensive, and are also associated with caveats ranging from primary and secondary perineural catheter failure to small additional risk of block site complications. Adjuvants present their own challenges and successful track records. One trial investigated the effect of dexamethasone added to ropivacaine for upper extremity fracture surgery. Patients in the group receiving ropivacaine plus dexamethasone had a longer block by 5 hours, and less peak pain after the block had worn off, as compared with those receiving plain bupivacaine only.[21] To interpret this study, we need to first consider that, in most of the patients, acute postoperative pain will decrease over the first hours and days after surgery.[22] So a longer block can simply "land" a patient on a point further down their pain trajectory, when pain has naturally subsided more, and the pain intensity is less. This study illustrates the somewhat confounding effects of dexamethasone—it may have prolonged the nerve block to a degree whereby the patient was naturally more pain-free than those patients who experienced a more abrupt resolution of the block 5 hours earlier. Moreover, the relative analgesic contributions of the peripheral, perineural and systemic effects of corticosteroid agents remain to be clarified. One study design that could potentially decrease such confusion is to have 3 groups, one with perineural dexamethasone, one with systemic dexamethasone, and one with plain local anesthetic.

Finally, a recent retrospective cohort study summarized 972 patients undergoing peripheral nerve blocks for ambulatory surgery, of whom approximately 50% had developed pain scores of ≥ 7 on the NRS scale after a previously well-performing block.[6] The authors reported that younger, female, orthopedic (bone surgery) patients, and those who did not receive intravenous dexamethasone, had a higher risk of rebound pain, but it should be noted that the odds ratios (OR) were between 0.98 and 1.82, suggesting that the development of rebound pain was likely multifactorial. Other factors identified in the machine learning part of the study were the choice of local anesthetic and the duration of motor block. This may reflect another variant of the above-mentioned hypothesis, that longer block duration by choosing longer acting drugs may, indeed, place patients in a more favorable position, and lead to decreased pain on block resolution.

PATIENT EXPECTATIONS

Pain perception involves both physical and emotional components. The quantification of rebound pain relies on patient-reported pain scores at various timepoints during the postoperative recovery. Patients who receive effective peripheral nerve blocks are at risk for comparison bias affecting their reported pain scores. Patients cannot help but compare their current pain to previous values as a benchmark. Psychological research has shown that negative stimuli are enhanced more significantly by strong contrasts and sudden changes, like in the case of a nerve block wearing off.[23] The environment may have pronounced effects as well. Experiencing acute pain in a highly monitored PACU with a high nursing-to-patient ratio and providers accustomed to managing acute pain and titrating analgesics in a timely fashion is far different than experiencing acute pain at home. Time of the day might also play an important role in pain perception, as physical and emotional distress are tolerated and coped with differently during daylight hours and at night. Additionally, it is relatively common for the block to be wearing off during nighttime because of the timing of the block during the day. Another important component mentioned above is the relative intensity of pain at rest and pain with movement that are strongly influenced by initial and surgical injuries, methods of immobilization, and physical therapy.

Patients expect postsurgical pain, and it is one of their most commonly reported surgical concerns.[24,25] It is unknown how those expectations are modified when they receive regional anesthesia, from preprocedural explanation to actual experience. Managing patient expectations of their postsurgical pain with nerve blocks may be critical, though understudied. The logical significance of a highly variable "reference point" for anticipated pain is also unknown. Patients who expect a pain-free and opioid-free surgical recovery are at risk of being disappointed especially if they are undergoing predictably painful procedures like shoulder arthroplasty. As part of the standard preprocedural nerve block evaluation and education, patients should be given a realistic expectation of block duration and understanding of the signs associated with block resolution. To date, when studied systematically, patient education materials about peripheral nerve blocks are highly variable and often written in sophisticated language that may not be fully comprehensible to some patients.[26] Educational initiatives such as preprocedural classes and meeting with anesthesiologists before the day of surgery have been shown to increase the rates at which patients accept regional anesthesia options, but have not been studied to determine if there is an effect on postoperative rebound pain.[27,28] It is also unclear if the patients understand the expected course of postsurgical pain following surgery as pain trajectories are also understudied and insufficiently understood by the health care providers themselves. Having a robust pain management plan to transition the patient from nerve block analgesia to oral analgesics will also likely mitigate the effects of rebound pain, though this has not been formally studied. There is no great understanding of the potentially beneficial effects of patients learning from their previous perioperative experiences on their expectations either. And finally, the roles of innate psychosocial patient characteristics such as catastrophizing and the placebo and nocebo phenomena in rebound pain occurrence and course are also unknown.

What about provider expectations? This field, abundant in anecdotes, is woefully unexplored, but also culturally difficult to study. What the members of the multidisciplinary care team expect from the patient and from each other may play a critical role in patient recovery, patient perceptions, and patient expectations. This is also the place to emphasize the importance of urgently and collaboratively assessing, discussing, and addressing symptoms and signs, including severe breakthrough pain, that is uncharacteristic and out of proportion! Failure to do so might lead *ad extremis* to missed or delayed diagnoses of life- and limb-threatening conditions such as acute compartment syndrome or more insidious complications such as postsurgical inflammatory neuropathy.

In conclusion, pain following the resolution of nerve blocks is quite common—in fact, it should be arguably expected after many surgical procedures. However, this does not automatically mean that patients should not be satisfied with their regional anesthetic. Ironfield and colleagues observed that more than 50% of patients reported moderate or severe pain after peripheral nerve block resolution, yet 94.7% of the patients reported that they would have a nerve block for future surgery.[12] Even in the subgroup of patients that reported severe pain after block resolution, 91.2% of patients would get a block again.[12] Then, should this be interpreted as a separate phenomenon or as a mere "wrinkle" in the postoperative analgesia planning to be improved upon?

Operationally, it will be important to distinguish severe postnerve block pain that has significant clinical effects from pain that is to be naturally expected with block resolution. It would be difficult to argue that a transitorily elevated pain score that is successfully managed with previously prescribed medications in trivial doses which also does not change overall patient satisfaction has any significant impact on postoperative recovery and overall outcomes. Therefore, only cases whereby patients are unable to have their care advanced due to high intravenous opioid requirements or need to be readmitted for pain management should be reviewed when designing effective strategies and interventions to mitigate rebound pain.

CLINICAL CONSEQUENCE

So where do we go from here? From the evidence obtained thus far, it seems that there is only a very modest theoretic underpinning to "rebound pain" as a separate and pathophysiologic entity. Yet, the contribution of potential pathologic processes, which may involve neurotoxic and local proinflammatory effects of local anesthetics, is unclear.[29,30] Meanwhile, it is evident that clinical studies consistently demonstrate high rates of moderate to severe pain after block resolution. So, in some way, we may be diminishing or even offsetting the positive effects of regional anesthetic techniques by not embedding them into a comprehensive perioperative multimodal analgesic regimen. Hamilton, in his recent editorial, rightfully alluded to the preconception that patients with a nerve block awaken pain-free, transition rapidly through or even bypass the PACU, and then end up on the floor or at home once the block wears off. This transition needs to be actively managed—the current deficits possibly being almost entirely due to the abrupt and somewhat disconnected switch of pain management "ownership" from anesthesia to surgery providers. Indeed, a collaborative multidisciplinary approach has been described by Saminiemi and colleagues as being successful in avoiding excessive pain on block resolution.[19]

So, should we call it just that, *pain on block resolution*? Another consideration in assigning a nomenclature to this problem is that it oversimplifies the clinical complexity we face in the operating rooms. It is more nuanced to discuss the benefits and risks of regional anesthesia with a view to aligning the pain management plan across services and into the postdischarge period, but it becomes quite easy to brush away regional anesthesia as a management option "... *because of all the rebound pain* ...". In that sense, the undersigned authors welcome and encourage research on improving the transition from nerve block to systemic pain management but would also argue against using "rebound pain" as terminology going forward. A term such as "post resolution pain" or "pain after block resolution" would be a more neutral designator for the time being, and until we better understand the etiology, scope, and gravity of the problem.

We join Munoz-Leyva,[1] Lavand'homme,[5] and Hamilton[7] in their call to emphasize the structured implementation of multimodal pain management as the primary strategy to prevent and mitigate pain after block resolution. One important facet discussed by Munoz-Leyva and colleagues was that pain after block resolution was typically reported after dense blockade (surgical anesthesia).[1] Some centers regularly avoid long-acting surgical anesthesia in patients if the block is not used as a primary anesthetic. The advantage of giving reduced concentrations, for example, bupivacaine 0.25% to supplement a general anesthetic is that severe pain should be reasonably controlled, but from the outset, concomitant nonopioid and opioid medication is often necessary, such that the patient never transitions from no pain (nor sensation, nor movement) to severe pain, but perhaps from mild to moderate pain, which would be tolerated better and managed more easily. Anecdotally, some patients are also often distressed by long-lasting surgical anesthesia following procedures. Yet, an alternative argument would emphasize that a decreased local anesthetic dose is also typically associated with a decreased block duration, with a higher likelihood of block resolution falling within a time period when the nociceptive input from the surgical/injury site is still intense enough to cause severe rebound pain. Another strategy is to use multimodal perineural techniques[31] or continuous techniques[32] to cover the period of expected intense pain sufficiently, though more research on expected pain trajectories for many procedures are needed. Lastly, education and management of patient (and provider) expectations play a substantial role in defining satisfaction after surgery. Therefore, improving the quality and availability of patient-centered educational materials, as well as proving vigilant and effective follow-up remain critical in ensuring that patients continue to thrive perioperatively with the benefits and appreciation of regional anesthesia.

CLINICS CARE POINTS

- When establishing a perioperative analgesic plan, patient-centered factors (eg, opioid use, biopsychosocial determinants), and procedure-specific characteristics (eg, how long do we expect severe pain to persist) need to be taken into account.
- Nerve blocks that predictably wear off before the strong pain has subsided can cause a resurgence in pain.
- We do not know at this point whether "rebound pain" is a distinct pathophysiological entity or a badly timed nerve block.
- Nerve blocks that predictably wear off before the strong pain has subsided need a comprehensive pain management transition strategy to assure a balanced transition to systemic analgesia.

ACKNOWLEDGMENTS

This manuscript was supported by the Departments by making academic time available.

REFERENCES

1. Munoz-Leyva F, Cubillos J, Chin KJ. Managing rebound pain after regional anesthesia. Korean J Anesthesiol 2020;73:372–83.
2. Williams BA, Bottegal MT, Kentor ML, et al. Rebound pain scores as a function of femoral nerve block duration after anterior cruciate ligament reconstruction: retrospective analysis of a prospective, randomized clinical trial. Reg Anesth Pain Med 2007;32:186–92.
3. Kolarczyk LM, Williams BA. Transient heat hyperalgesia during resolution of ropivacaine sciatic nerve block in the rat. Reg Anesth Pain Med 2011;36:220–4.
4. Galos DK, Taormina DP, Crespo A, et al. Does Brachial Plexus Blockade Result in Improved Pain Scores After Distal Radius Fracture Fixation? A Randomized Trial. Clin Orthop Relat Res 2016;474:1247–54.
5. Lavand'homme P. Rebound pain after regional anesthesia in the ambulatory patient. Curr Opin Anaesthesiol 2018;31:679–84.

6. Barry GS, Bailey JG, Sardinha J, et al. Factors associated with rebound pain after peripheral nerve block for ambulatory surgery. Br J Anaesth 2021;126:862–71.

7. Hamilton DL. Rebound pain: distinct pain phenomenon or nonentity? Br J Anaesth 2021;126:761–3.

8. Woo JH, Lee HJ, Oh HW, et al. Perineural dexamethasone reduces rebound pain after ropivacaine single injection interscalene block for arthroscopic shoulder surgery: a randomized controlled trial. Reg Anesth Pain Med 2021;46:965–70.

9. Dada O, Gonzalez Zacarias A, Ongaigui C, et al. Does rebound pain after peripheral nerve block for orthopedic surgery impact postoperative analgesia and opioid consumption? a narrative review. Int J Environ Res Public Health 2019; 16:3257.

10. Henningsen MJ, Sort R, Moller AM, et al. Peripheral nerve block in ankle fracture surgery: a qualitative study of patients' experiences. Anaesthesia 2018;73:49–58.

11. Sort R, Brorson S, Gogenur I, et al. Rebound pain following peripheral nerve block anaesthesia in acute ankle fracture surgery: An exploratory pilot study. Acta Anaesthesiol Scand 2019;63:396–402.

12. Ironfield CM, Barrington MJ, Kluger R, et al. Are patients satisfied after peripheral nerve blockade? Results from an International Registry of Regional Anesthesia. Reg Anesth Pain Med 2014;39:48–55.

13. Hamilton GM, Ramlogan R, Lui A, et al. Peripheral Nerve Blocks for Ambulatory Shoulder Surgery: A Population-based Cohort Study of Outcomes and Resource Utilization. Anesthesiology 2019;131:1254–63.

14. Janda A, Lydic R, Welch KB, et al. Thermal hyperalgesia after sciatic nerve block in rat is transient and clinically insignificant. Reg Anesth Pain Med 2013;38: 151–4.

15. An K, Elkassabany NM, Liu J. Dexamethasone as adjuvant to bupivacaine prolongs the duration of thermal antinociception and prevents bupivacaine-induced rebound hyperalgesia via regional mechanism in a mouse sciatic nerve block model. PLoS One 2015;10:e0123459.

16. Williams BA, Hough KA, Tsui BY, et al. Neurotoxicity of adjuvants used in perineural anesthesia and analgesia in comparison with ropivacaine. Reg Anesth Pain Med 2011;36:225–30.

17. Kissin I. Preemptive analgesia. Anesthesiology 2000;93:1138–43.

18. Goldstein RY, Montero N, Jain SK, et al. Efficacy of popliteal block in postoperative pain control after ankle fracture fixation: a prospective randomized study. J Orthop Trauma 2012;26:557–61.

19. Samineni AV, Seaver T, Sing DC, et al. Peripheral nerve blocks associated with shorter length of stay without increasing readmission rate for ankle open reduction internal fixation in the outpatient setting: a propensity-matched analysis. J Foot Ankle Surg 2021. https://doi.org/10.1053/j.jfas.2021.10.017.

20. Hade AD, Okano S, Pelecanos A, et al. Factors associated with low levels of patient satisfaction following peripheral nerve block. Anaesth Intensive Care 2021; 49:125–32.

21. Fang J, Shi Y, Du F, et al. The effect of perineural dexamethasone on rebound pain after ropivacaine single-injection nerve block: a randomized controlled trial. BMC Anesthesiol 2021;21:47.

22. Panzenbeck P, von Keudell A, Joshi GP, et al. Procedure-specific acute pain trajectory after elective total hip arthroplasty: systematic review and data synthesis. Br J Anaesth 2021;127:110–32.

23. Voichek G, Novemsky N. Asymmetric Hedonic Contrast: Pain Is More Contrast Dependent Than Pleasure. Psychol Sci 2021;32:1038–46.

24. Gan TJ, Habib AS, Miller TE, et al. Incidence, patient satisfaction, and perceptions of post-surgical pain: results from a US national survey. Curr Med Res Opin 2014;30:149–60.
25. Berkowitz R, Vu J, Brummett C, et al. The Impact of Complications and Pain on Patient Satisfaction. Ann Surg 2021;273:1127–34.
26. Kumar G, Howard SK, Kou A, et al. Availability and Readability of Online Patient Education Materials Regarding Regional Anesthesia Techniques for Perioperative Pain Management. Pain Med 2017;18:2027–32.
27. Brooks BS, Barman J, Ponce BA, et al. An electronic surgical order, undertaking patient education, and obtaining informed consent for regional analgesia before the day of surgery reduce block-related delays. Local Reg Anesth 2016;9:59–64.
28. Elkassabany NM, Abraham D, Huang S, et al. Patient education and anesthesia choice for total knee arthroplasty. Patient Educ Couns 2017;100:1709–13.
29. Verlinde M, Hollmann MW, Stevens MF, et al. Local Anesthetic-Induced Neurotoxicity. Int J Mol Sci 2016;17:339.
30. Gordon SM, Chuang BP, Wang XM, et al. The differential effects of bupivacaine and lidocaine on prostaglandin E2 release, cyclooxygenase gene expression and pain in a clinical pain model. Anesth Analg 2008;106:321–7, table of contents.
31. Williams BA, Butt MT, Zeller JR, et al. Multimodal perineural analgesia with combined bupivacaine-clonidine-buprenorphine-dexamethasone: safe in vivo and chemically compatible in solution. Pain Med 2015;16:186–98.
32. Ilfeld BM. Continuous peripheral nerve blocks: a review of the published evidence. Anesth Analg 2011;113:904–25.

Multimodal Analgesia

Archana O'Neill, MD, Philipp Lirk, MD, PhD*

KEYWORDS

- Multimodal analgesia • Preventive analgesia • Peripheral sensitization
- Central sensitization • Persistent postsurgical pain • Opioid-induced hyperalgesia
- Local infiltration analgesia • Nerve block

KEY POINTS

- Moderate to severe pain continues to be frequent after surgery.
- Analgesia needs to strike a balance between adequate pain relief and facilitation of early mobilization and discharge.
- Multimodal analgesia is the balanced application of low to moderate doses of nonopioids, ideally in combination, to maximize analgesic activity and minimize the risk of side effects.

INTRODUCTION

Inadequate perioperative pain is, unfortunately, frequent, and has clinically relevant consequences, including decreased patient satisfaction, delayed postoperative mobilization, development of chronic postoperative pain, a higher likelihood of experiencing cardiac and pulmonary complications, and increased morbidity and mortality.[1] Impediments to postoperative mobilization are especially harmful in orthopedic surgery as better outcomes have been clearly demonstrated in patients who begin ambulating more quickly.[2] However, orthopedic surgery is, in general, one the most painful types of surgery performed.[3]

Pain and its sequelae cause enormous personal and economic problems, and in the United States, Acute and Chronic pain account for greater health care expenditures than heart disease, diabetes, and cancer combined.[4] Yet, a solution is more difficult than anticipated: in an attempt to improve awareness of the necessity of adequate pain management was through the designation of pain as the "fifth vital sign" in the 1990s by the American Pain Society (APS), which was met with great initial enthusiasm worldwide.[5,6] In the subsequent years, the prescription of opioids climbed to unprecedented levels, especially in the United States, Canada and Australia (it had been

Department of Anesthesiology, Perioperative and Pain Medicine, Brigham and Women's Hospital, Harvard Medical School, 75 Francis Street, Boston, MA 02115, USA
* Corresponding author. Department of Anesthesiology, Perioperative and Pain Medicine, Brigham and Women's Hospital, Harvard Medical School, 75 Francis Street, Boston, MA 02115.
E-mail address: plirk@bwh.harvard.edu

Anesthesiology Clin 40 (2022) 455–468
https://doi.org/10.1016/j.anclin.2022.04.002
1932-2275/22/© 2022 Elsevier Inc. All rights reserved.

climbing slowly before, truth to be told).[7] So in the meantime, many Institutions central to United States medicine, including the American Medical Association, the Joint Commission, and the Centers for Medicare and Medicaid services have abandoned advocacy for "the fifth vital sign." If we take pain scores reported in the context of clinical trials as a reflection of clinical success, there has not been a real improvement in the treatment of acute postoperative pain,[8] and looking at the clinical side of things gives an equally pessimistic view: inadequately treated pain is still frequent even after so-called minor procedures,[1] and 30% to 80% of patients continue to report moderate to severe pain immediately after surgery.[9,10]

Why is it so difficult to achieve adequate postoperative analgesia? Adequacy of pain treatment depends on multiple factors related to the procedure,[11] patient factors,[12] and available (and feasible) treatment techniques. The medications available to treat pain effectively include opioids and nonopioids. Even though opioids are still widely used,[13] more information on their misuse, limitations, and side effects is becoming available, including the risk of dependence and opioid-induced hyperalgesia (OIH).[6] Even though calls have been made to implement opioid-free anesthesia, there is currently insufficient evidence that true opioid-free anesthesia would be appropriate on a broad scale, unless it is based on long-acting or continuous regional block techniques. For most patients, a balanced multimodal analgesic regimen with opioids limited to the minimum necessary for the shortest period possible seems to be the best evidence-based way ahead.[7] The goals of multimodal analgesia are to attack pain from several sides, to achieve the optimal balance between treatment effect and side effects, and to wean the patient off opioids as soon as possible. This article provides an introduction to the systemic medications frequently used in multimodal analgesia, as well as the use of local infiltration analgesia (LIA) in orthopedic surgery.

MULTIMODAL ANALGESIA

Multimodal analgesia has been defined as the use of 2 or more analgesics or techniques that target different mechanisms or pathways in the nociceptive system.[14] The combination of several drugs in the repertoire allows for lower doses of each individual drugs, thereby lowering the side effects of each individual drug, while preserving overall efficacy.[15,16] This result should, in theory, translate to improved analgesia, enhanced functional recovery and reduced opioid-related adverse effects.[17] The American Society of Anesthesiologists (ASA), the American Pain Society (APS) and the American Society of Regional Anesthesia and Pain Medicine (ASRA) have strongly encouraged the use of multimodal analgesia in the management of acute pain in the perioperative setting,[18,19] and it is now considered the standard of care for all postsurgical patients.[13] Orthopedic surgery has also embraced multimodal analgesia for at least a decade due to the pain associated with these procedures,[3] and multimodal analgesia has resulted in better analgesic outcomes in this type of surgery.[20] In addition, enhanced recovery after surgery (ERAS) protocols focus heavily on the use of multimodal analgesia with opioid-sparing techniques.[21] These types of protocols are also being implemented in orthopedic surgery with a focus on total joint replacement which further highlights the need for good multimodal strategies to optimize outcomes in these patients.[22] However, despite the overwhelming evidence, and the practice guidelines, some of which have been around for a decade,[18] and wide array of available interventions, there is still considerable heterogeneity in the practice of multimodal analgesia.[13] The following paragraphs detail the systemic analgesics available for patient- and procedure-specific pain management. They are grouped into classical nonopioid analgesics, adjuvant analgesics, and LIA.

Classical Nonopioid Drugs

Acetaminophen (paracetamol)

Acetaminophen is one of the older and most prescribed medications in the world with a long track record of use as an analgesic and antipyretic and a very favorable safety profile.[23] Despite its use for decades, the exact mechanism of action is still unclear, and the therapeutic targets conjectured include the central splice variant cyclo-oxygenase (COX-3), the endogenous opioid and descending inhibitory serotoninergic system, the nitric oxide synthase, and the endocannabinoid system.[23,24] The most prominent potential adverse effect of acetaminophen is severe hepatotoxicity, which is caused by the toxic metabolite, N-acetyl-p-benzoquinone imine (NAPQI). This toxicity is caused by absolute overdosing, or failure to take into account preexisting liver damage (increased cytochrome P450 activation, decreased availability of glutathione, and chronic severe alcohol abuse).[25] Even though adequate therapeutic doses of the medication do not seem to exacerbate stable chronic liver disease, total daily dosing should be reduced, and duration of use should be minimized in these situations.[23]

Several meta-analyses have confirmed that paracetamol can reduce opioid consumption by 20%[26,27] with a very good perioperative side effect profile. Furthermore, there is valuable evidence to support the efficacy of acetaminophen use in conjunction with another nonopioid adjunct such as an NSAID or COX-2 inhibitor to improve postoperative analgesia and reduce opioid consumption.[28,29] Acetaminophen should be a key component of multimodal perioperative pain management and can be used in persons with gastrointestinal disorders, renal disease or advanced age.[30] But what if the patient has no contraindications to NSAID? Thybo and colleagues in the PANSAID trial answered this question by showing that in patients undergoing total hip arthroplasty, adding NSAID (in this case, ibuprofen) to paracetamol improved analgesia, whereas adding paracetamol to ibuprofen did not.[31] This may indicate that the major analgesic effect of the combination between paracetamol and NSAID lies with the NSAID, at least in orthopedic surgery.

Nonsteroidal anti-inflammatory drugs and COX-2 inhibitors

Nonsteroidal antiinflammatory drugs (NSAIDs) and COX-2 inhibitors are useful drugs with antiinflammatory, antipyretic, and analgesic properties.[32] NSAIDs, both nonselective and selective, are useful analgesics as they inhibit inflammation, one of the main sources of postoperative pain. They are part of the multimodal recommendations by ASA, APS, and ASRA, and should be used whenever feasible.[18,19] Several meta-analyses have highlighted their potential to improve analgesia and reduce opioid-induced side effects.[28,33] NSAIDs or COX-2 inhibitors were also found to have specific efficacy in total joint arthroplasty.[34] Furthermore, as NSAIDs are known to provide effective analgesia for musculoskeletal pain and the data for NSAIDs delaying bone healing remains inconclusive, the recently published Clinical Practice Guidelines for Pain Management in Acute Musculoskeletal Injury now strongly supports the routine use of NSAIDs as part of the multimodal analgesic plan for both operative and nonoperative fracture care.[35] In summary, the choice of NSAIDs and COX-2 inhibitor medication should be guided by surgical factors as well as patient comorbidities. Recognizing the potential for complications and in the absence of contraindications, a brief judicious perioperative course of NSAIDs or COX inhibitors should be considered safe in most settings.

Adjuvant Analgesics

Glucocorticoids/dexamethasone

Dexamethasone is routinely used by anesthesiologists to minimize postoperative nausea and vomiting (PONV),[36] and glucocorticoids are also well known for their antiinflammatory effects and ability to reduce tissue injury. Their analgesic properties stem from their ability to reduce prostaglandin synthesis through the inhibition of phospholipase enzyme and COX-2, thereby decreasing the proinflammatory output from the cyclooxygenase and lipoxygenase pathways.[37,38] Dexamethasone has been studied in the prevention of pain, but not in the treatment of established pain. De Oliveira showed that the dose of dexamethasone needed to achieve decreased pain scores postoperatively was 0.2 mg/kg, whereas 0.1 mg/kg was not effective.[39] Another review suggested 8 mg as the commonly used dose to achieve pain reduction.[40] Another study found that intravenous dexamethasone was also effective in prolonging time to first analgesic after surgery under spinal anesthesia.[41] One surgery in which efficacy seems particularly valuable is spine surgery, whereby 8 mg of dexamethasone reduced postoperative pain without increasing side effects.[38]

One argument against perioperative dexamethasone administration is the risk of hyperglycemia, but a recent retrospective study on 4800 orthopedic surgery patients showed that the risk was small, and very likely more than outweighed by shorter length of stay.[42] Dexamethasone is an inexpensive and easily administered medication frequently used in the perioperative period for PONV prophylaxis and should be part of multimodal regimens unless contraindicated.

Gabapentinoids
Gabapentin was originally introduced as an anticonvulsant in the 1990s, followed by pregabalin, which featured improved oral pharmacokinetics and a longer half-life.[43] Over time, there was increased off-label use for perioperative analgesia, and indeed, several meta-analyses supported the usefulness of gabapentinoids in reducing acute postoperative pain and opioid consumption.[43–45] The 2016 guidelines by the APS, ASA, and ASRA still advocated for the use of gabapentinoids as a component of multimodal analgesia preoperatively as a strong recommendation with moderate quality evidence.[19] However, since then, more critical studies have emerged, highlighting the risk of respiratory depression if combined with opioids,[46] and dizziness.[47] The FDA issued a warning regarding the use of gabapentinoids with opioids in December 2019, and more recent reviews and advisories no longer advocate for the administration of gabapentinoids on a broad scale.[48] Therefore, many contemporary Institutions have stopped the protocolized perioperative administration of gabapentinoids, unless patients are already taking them, or there are specific concerns. One remaining argument for gabapentinoids might be that there was a suggestion of decreased chronic pain and decreased chronic opioid use with perioperative gabapentin,[49] but these findings would need confirmation. For the moment, after almost 20 years of enthusiasm and research focus, the broad perioperative use of gabapentinoids seems to come to an end.

N-methyl-ᴅ-aspartate antagonists
The perioperative relevance of N-methyl-ᴅ-aspartate (NMDA) receptors lies in their pivotal role in central sensitization caused by peripheral nociceptive stimulation, and NMDA antagonists can be both preventive and therapeutic against sensitization.[50] The NMDA receptor has also been implicated in persistent postoperative pain, hypersensitivity, windup, and allodynia, opioid-induced tolerance, and OIH.[51] The 2 most relevant drugs in clinical use are ketamine and magnesium.

Ketamine. Ketamine is one of the older drugs in our armamentarium having first been developed in the 1960s as an anesthetic agent with analgesic properties.[51] Ketamine has a wide variety of actions, including effects on μ-opioid receptors, muscarinic receptors, monoaminergic receptors, γ-aminobutyric acid receptors, and multiple others.[51,52] However, its principle pharmacologic function is antagonism at NMDA receptors. In that sense, it is a rather nonspecific drug that works relatively weakly on a wide array of targets. One could say, the exact counterpart to high-affinity drugs such as remifentanil. Its main effects are anesthetic and analgesic at higher doses (bolus of 0.5–1 mg/kg), or anti-hyperalgesic at lower doses (slow bolus of 0.1 mg/kg, typically followed by low-dose infusion of 0.1 mg/kg/h). Ketamine use is increasing in the clinical area, not least as a result of the opioid crisis in parts of the Western world.[53] Consensus guidelines by ASRA, AAPM, and ASA were published in 2018, and they noted that subanesthetic doses of ketamine exhibited the most benefit in surgeries associated with significant postoperative pain such as thoracic surgery, upper and lower abdominal surgery, and orthopedic (both limb and spine) surgery.[52,54] Procedures which cause mild levels of pain, and are carried out in opioid-naïve patients do not warrant routine perioperative ketamine administration.[54]

In addition to the type of surgery, some patient indications for ketamine treatment exist with the most compelling being an opioid-tolerant or opioid-dependent patient.[54] Although there is some conflicting evidence regarding this indication, a 2010 study by Loftus and colleagues (N = 102) [55] and a more recent 2019 study by Boenigk and colleagues (N = 129)[56] both demonstrated that postoperative opioid consumption was reduced in opioid-dependent and opioid-tolerant patients that received ketamine infusions perioperatively. The consensus statement mentioned above also concluded that there is at least mild benefit and more likely moderate benefit of subanesthetic dosing of perioperative ketamine for this particular patient population.[52] Other target populations include patients with sleep apnea.[52,57]

In terms of the dose range considered subanesthetic but still effective for acute pain, lower doses should be given preference over higher doses. Specifically, the consensus committee recommends limiting a bolus of ketamine to 0.35 mg/kg and infusions for acute pain to 1 mg/kg/h to provide effective analgesia while minimizing adverse reactions.[52] We suggest starting even lower, at 0.1 to 0.15 mg/kg as a bolus and 0.1 mg/kg/h as an infusion, and to titrate upward, with the main goal being the avoidance of side effects. This would be in line with the results of the 2018 PODCAST trial, which showed a greater incidence of hallucinations and nightmares with escalating doses of ketamine.[58] Of note, that study did not find an analgesic effect of a single large bolus of ketamine in patients 60 years or older undergoing major surgery.[58]

The contraindications are mostly related to the side effects of ketamine, and include uncontrolled cardiovascular disease, pregnancy, and psychosis.[52] Ketamine should be used with caution in patients with moderate hepatic disease and avoided in patients with severe liver disease, that is, cirrhosis.[52] Elevated intracranial pressure or intraocular pressure also precludes the safe use of ketamine from the available evidence,[52] but these recommendations most often refer to high-dose administration. Data on the potential of ketamine to decrease persistent postsurgical pain (PPSP) are inconclusive at this point.[59]

Magnesium. Magnesium has been studied for decades in the context of anesthesia due to its central depressant effects, but more recently, the focus has shifted to its utility in perioperative analgesia stemming from its known antagonism of NDMA receptors and role in preventing central sensitization. Tramer and colleagues first described the analgesic properties of perioperative magnesium,[60] and this has been validated by subsequent trials and meta-analyses.[61–64] Dosing can be either in the form of a bolus or an infusion intraoperatively with it typically ranging from 30 to 50 mg/kg for the bolus and infusion rates of 8 to 15 mg/kg/h[65] Furthermore, magnesium has a wide therapeutic window and a good safety profile when used at therapeutic doses, although patients should be monitored closely for signs of hypermagnesemia, especially with renal insufficiency.[66]

Alpha-2 agonists

The widespread use of α-2 agonists is grounded in their pharmacologic actions, including sedation, anxiolysis, hypnosis, sympatholysis, and analgesia, with no respiratory depression.[67] Mechanisms of action include T hyperpolarization of supraspinal noradrenergic neurons which decreases neuronal firing in the locus coeruleus and leads to an inhibition of sympathetic neurotransmitter release and suppression of activity in descending sympathetic pathways and is responsible for the sedative properties of these drugs.[68][Grewal, 2011 #4221] Dexmedetomidine and Clonidine are the 2 most frequently used α-2 agonists perioperatively.

Clonidine. Clonidine can be used pre, intra, or postoperatively, including in children.[68] It has different routes of administration, including intravenous, perineural, neuraxial, and transdermal. It is also useful as an anesthesia and analgesia adjuvant and has been shown to decrease MAC requirements as well as a valuable additive to local anesthetics for regional techniques.[68] Clonidine is an analgesic and opioid-sparing drug.[67]

The results of the POISE-2 study (2014) suggested that the routine administration of clonidine was associated with a greater risk of clinically significant hypotension and nonfatal cardiac arrest without improving cardiac outcomes in patients undergoing noncardiac surgery.[69] The main lesson for us, therefore, is to use good judgment on when to administer clonidine, weighing risks and benefits, and being ready to treat hypotension when it ensues. Other indications are patients at risk of alcohol withdrawal,[70] excess anxiety,[71] or postoperative shivering.[72] Usual doses for the latter indications are 0.5 mcg/kg body weight, except for shivering, whereby 0.25 to 0.3 mcg/kg can be used as a starting dose.

Dexmedetomidine. Dexmedetomidine was approved by the FDA in 1999 as an analgesic and sedative medication in the intensive care setting (ICU) setting.[68] It is a much more highly selective α-2 agonist compared with clonidine, and its half-life is about 2 hours versus 9 to 12 hours for clonidine. Because the α-2$_A$ receptor subtype is relevant for pain, it may be better analgesic than clonidine. Several meta-analyses have examined the effectiveness of these α-2 agonists in postoperative analgesia. One such meta-analysis included 30 studies (N = 1792), with 933 receiving either clonidine or dexmedetomidine, and the authors concluded that perioperative systemic alpha-2 agonists reduced postoperative opioid consumption (down 30% compared with placebo), pain intensity, and nausea without prolonging recovery times,[67] while the most common adverse effects noted were bradycardia and arterial hypotension.[67] Martinez *and colleagues* found that α-2 agonists were similar to NSAIDs and COX-2 inhibitors in reducing opioid consumption, analgesia, and PONV, and superior to acetaminophen alone.[28] Other meta-analyses have similarly described decreased postoperative pain and reduced opioid consumption as well as other secondary outcomes such as reduced opioid related adverse effects and PONV.[73–75] Dexmedetomidine seems to be especially useful in spine surgery, intracranial neurosurgery, and bariatric surgery.[75–77] The reader is alerted to the fact that clonidine and dexmedetomidine have been accused of causing false-positive pathologic readings during neuromonitoring of spinal motor pathways,[78] but this finding has not been reliably replicated and different institutions may have specific policies in place regarding dexmedetomidine and its place in neurosurgery when monitoring is used. Based on its ability to reduce both anesthetic and opioid requirements intraoperatively, dexmedetomidine seems to be a valuable tool in ERAS protocols and has significantly improved postoperative outcomes in this context.[79]

Intravenous administration of dexmedetomidine is most common, and dosing typically consists of a bolus dose between 0.25 and 1 mcg/kg given over 10 minutes and infusion rates between 0.2 and 0.6 mcg/kg/h. The bolus dose may be omitted in patients with tenuous hemodynamics. Due to its hemodynamic effects, dexmedetomidine should be administered in monitored settings, such as the OR, PACU, or ICU. Initial dose when used for analgesic purposes should be limited to 0.5 mcg/kg body weight.

Local Infiltration Analgesia

Local infiltration analgesia (LIA) encompasses the instillation of local anesthetics and other adjuvant medications directly around surgical sites by the surgeon. Although this practice had been performed in multiple types of procedures and different settings for some time, the practice of LIA in orthopedic surgery was brought to the forefront in 2008 by Kerr and Kohan who developed a technique for pain management in total hip and knee replacement by infiltrating a mix of long acting local anesthetic (ropivacaine), epinephrine, and an NSAID (ketorolac) into the tissues around the surgical field to improve analgesia without significant side effects.[80] Their case study of 325 patients with total hip replacement (THR) and total knee replacement (TKR) demonstrated overall relatively low pain scores (NRS 0–3), no morphine usage in two-thirds of patients, and early ambulation as well as early discharge for about 70% of patients.[80] This new technique was thought to be particularly useful in the context of lower extremity joint replacement due to its ease of performance and ability to provide adequate analgesia, without lower extremity weakness, leading to earlier mobilization and improved functional recovery, a top priority to avoid complications such as deep venous thrombosis, infection, and hardware malfunction.[80,81]

Since 2008, there have been numerous investigations on the efficacy of LIA in total joint replacement. In both THR and TKR, many different regional techniques including epidural, femoral nerve block (FNB), sciatic nerve block (SNB), lumbar plexus block (LPB), and fascia iliaca block (FIB) have also been studied to find the optimal analgesic regimen for each of these procedures.

Recently published guidelines for postoperative pain management in THR by the PROSPECT group found that LIA or FIB is beneficial as part of a multimodal analgesic plan, especially when other components of the multimodal regimen are contraindicated or when patients are at risk for increased postoperative pain, but other regional techniques such as epidural, FNB, and LPB are not recommended as adverse effects outweigh benefits.[82] These comprehensive guidelines were updated from 2010 guidelines which did not include LIA as part of the recommended multimodal regimen due to conflicting evidence, however, as more recent investigations have demonstrated a benefit from single injection LIA, it could be considered in THR.[82]

For TKR, controversy still remains regarding the most favorable analgesic regimen. As with THR, the goals of postoperative recovery after this procedure focus on optimizing analgesia to enhance early mobilization thereby improving recovery, speeding discharge, avoiding postoperative complications, and increasing patient satisfaction.[83] Over the years, numerous different techniques and regimens have been used with varying degrees of success. In 2014, Andersen and Kehlet established that LIA was beneficial as part of a multimodal analgesic plan for TKR compared with placebo for the initial postoperative period demonstrating decreased pain and reduction in opioid usage in the early (<48h) postoperative period.[84] Several years later, in 2017, a large network meta-analysis of 170 randomized controlled trials (RCTs) including

12,530 patients, found that a combined femoral and sciatic nerve block was the best technique overall to achieve decreased pain at rest, reduced opioid consumption, and best passive range of motion.[85] The take-home message from this very large meta-analysis was that blocking multiple nerves was superior to blocking a single nerve, LIA, or epidural analgesia when looking at those specific outcomes.[85] However, these peripheral nerve block techniques have several drawbacks as well, most importantly lower extremity motor weakness, which can impede early mobilization and lead to falls.[86]

Since early mobilization, adequate pain control, and decreased length of hospital stay are all important goals after TKR that need to be balanced, there has been a shift away from lower extremity nerve blocks, such as femoral nerve blocks, that lead to decreased mobility toward LIA and other nerve block techniques, such as the adductor canal block (ACB) which causes minimal to no lower extremity weakness and, in turn, lower chance of falls.[87–89] There have been multiple studies undertaken to examine whether LIA, ACB, or a combination of both is the most beneficial regimen for patients undergoing TKR with conflicting results. When answering this question, several factors need to be put more precisely: the first is the timepoint of assessment. For example, directly after emerging from TKR under general anesthesia supplemented with nerve blocks, femoral nerve block would give reasonable coverage of the surgical scar, and the anterior portion of the knee, whereas the adductor canal block by itself would typically not (as the scar extends more proximally than the area covered by the saphenous nerve). However, a couple of hours later, as the dermal nociceptive pain decreases and the deeper pain in the anterior compartment becomes more relevant, adductor canal blockade is a very powerful option to provide analgesia. LIA lasts for up to 18 to 24 hours, so the value of a single shot ACB is unclear, whereas pain on ambulation one to 2 days after surgery was lowest in a cohort receiving continuous adductor canal blockade.[90] Also, considerations depend on the hospital infrastructure, discharge planning, and standard operating practices. Whereas LIA has largely replaced nerve blocks as the primary analgesic pillar, many other regions of the world, including Europe, still place a much higher emphasis on nerve blocks as the bedrock of analgesia after TKR.

SUMMARY

The past decade has seen a dramatic shift from opioid-based analgesic methods to methods based primarily on nonopioids. We are now prioritizing regional anesthesia, LIA, and analgesic adjuvants over opioids and have learned that judicious patient- and procedure-specific use of multimodal drug regimens can achieve equal or better pain control with less side effects compared with opioid-based analgesia. Multimodal analgesia should be standard of care and used in all patients requiring systemic analgesia.

CLINICS CARE POINTS

- The components of the multimodal analgesic plan need to be tailored to procedure and patient (eg, specific drug contraindications).
- Pending there are no contraindications, baseline analgesia should include acetaminophen and either a nonsteroidal antiinflammatory agent (NSAID) or cyclo-oxygenase-2 inhibitor.
- The next step is to add adjuvants, such as dexamethasone, gabapentinoids, ketamine, and alpha-2-agonists. Dexamethasone has strong antiinflammatory properties. Gabapentinoids were highly popular for the last 20 years, but recent aggregated evidence suggests they are

less effective than once thought and may lead to more side effects, especially when initiated perioperatively. Ketamine should be initiated at very low doses, and increased in dose gradually, with the main goal of avoiding psychotropic side effects. Alpha-2-agonists may be especially useful in anxious patients.

- Local infiltration analgesia (LIA) has gained widespread scientific and clinical acceptance for total knee arthroplasty, its role in total hip or shoulder arthroplasty is subordinate.

ACKNOWLEDGMENTS

The current work was supported by the Department of Anesthesia by offering academic time.

DISCLOSURE

A. O'Neill: None. P. Lirk: None.

REFERENCES

1. Gerbershagen HJ, Aduckathil S, van Wijck AJ, et al. Pain intensity on the first day after surgery: a prospective cohort study comparing 179 surgical procedures. Anesthesiology 2013;118:934–44.
2. Sardana V, Burzynski JM, Scuderi GR. Adductor canal block or local infiltrate analgesia for pain control after total knee arthroplasty? A systematic review and meta-analysis of randomized controlled trials. J Arthroplasty 2019;34:183–9.
3. Pitchon DN, Dayan AC, Schwenk ES, et al. Updates on multimodal analgesia for orthopedic surgery. Anesthesiol Clin 2018;36:361–73.
4. Kharasch ED, Avram MJ, Clark JD. Rational perioperative opioid management in the era of the opioid crisis: reply. Anesthesiology 2020;133:942–3.
5. Levy N, Sturgess J, Mills P. Pain as the fifth vital sign" and dependence on the "numerical pain scale" is being abandoned in the US: Why? Br J Anaesth 2018; 120:435–8.
6. Wu CL, Raja SN. Treatment of acute postoperative pain. Lancet 2011;377: 2215–25.
7. Lirk P, Rathmell JP. Opioid-free anaesthesia: Con: it is too early to adopt opioid-free anaesthesia today. Eur J Anaesthesiol 2019;36:250–4.
8. Correll DJ, Vlassakov KV, Kissin I. No evidence of real progress in treatment of acute pain, 1993-2012: scientometric analysis. J Pain Res 2014;7:199–210.
9. Meissner W, Zaslansky R. A survey of postoperative pain treatments and unmet needs. Best Pract Res Clin Anaesthesiol 2019;33:269–86.
10. Gan TJ, Habib AS, Miller TE, et al. Incidence, patient satisfaction, and perceptions of post-surgical pain: results from a US national survey. Curr Med Res Opin 2014;30:149–60.
11. Joshi GP, Kehlet H, Group PW. Guidelines for perioperative pain management: need for re-evaluation. Br J Anaesth 2017;119:703–6.
12. Schreiber KL, Zinboonyahgoon N, Xu X, et al. Preoperative Psychosocial and Psychophysical Phenotypes as Predictors of Acute Pain Outcomes After Breast Surgery. J Pain 2018;20(5):540–56.
13. Ladha KS, Patorno E, Huybrechts KF, et al. Variations in the use of perioperative multimodal analgesic therapy. Anesthesiology 2016;124:837–45.
14. Manworren RC. Multimodal pain management and the future of a personalized medicine approach to pain. AORN J 2015;101:308–14.

15. Buvanendran A, Kroin JS. Multimodal analgesia for controlling acute postoperative pain. Curr Opin Anaesthesiol 2009;22:588–93.
16. Kehlet H, Dahl JB. The value of "multimodal" or "balanced analgesia" in postoperative pain treatment. Anesth Analg 1993;77:1048–56.
17. Buvanendran A, Kroin JS. Useful adjuvants for postoperative pain management. Best Pract Res Clin Anaesthesiol 2007;21:31–49.
18. American Society of Anesthesiologists Task Force on Acute Pain M. Practice guidelines for acute pain management in the perioperative setting: an updated report by the American Society of Anesthesiologists Task Force on Acute Pain Management. Anesthesiology 2012;116:248–73.
19. Chou R, Gordon DB, de Leon-Casasola OA, et al. Management of Postoperative Pain: A Clinical Practice Guideline From the American Pain Society, the American Society of Regional Anesthesia and Pain Medicine, and the American Society of Anesthesiologists' Committee on Regional Anesthesia, Executive Committee, and Administrative Council. J Pain 2016;17:131–57.
20. Halawi MJ, Grant SA, Bolognesi MP. Multimodal Analgesia for Total Joint Arthroplasty. Orthopedics 2015;38:e616–25.
21. Joshi GP, Kehlet H. Enhanced Recovery Pathways: Looking Into the Future. Anesth Analg 2019;128:5–7.
22. Frassanito L, Vergari A, Nestorini R, et al. Enhanced recovery after surgery (ERAS) in hip and knee replacement surgery: description of a multidisciplinary program to improve management of the patients undergoing major orthopedic surgery. Musculoskelet Surg 2020;104:87–92.
23. Oscier CD, Milner QJ. Peri-operative use of paracetamol. Anaesthesia 2009;64: 65–72.
24. Klinger-Gratz PP, Ralvenius WT, Neumann E, et al. Acetaminophen relieves inflammatory pain through cb1 cannabinoid receptors in the rostral ventromedial medulla. J Neurosci 2018;38:322–34.
25. Mattia C, Coluzzi F. What anesthesiologists should know about paracetamol (acetaminophen). Minerva Anestesiol 2009;75:644–53.
26. Remy C, Marret E, Bonnet F. Effects of acetaminophen on morphine side-effects and consumption after major surgery: meta-analysis of randomized controlled trials. Br J Anaesth 2005;94:505–13.
27. Toms L, McQuay HJ, Derry S, et al. Single dose oral paracetamol (acetaminophen) for postoperative pain in adults. Cochrane Database Syst Rev 2008;CD004602.
28. Martinez V, Beloeil H, Marret E, et al. Non-opioid analgesics in adults after major surgery: systematic review with network meta-analysis of randomized trials. Br J Anaesth 2017;118:22–31.
29. Ong CK, Seymour RA, Lirk P, et al. Combining paracetamol (acetaminophen) with nonsteroidal antiinflammatory drugs: a qualitative systematic review of analgesic efficacy for acute postoperative pain. Anesth Analg 2010;110:1170–9.
30. Joshi GP, Van de Velde M, Kehlet H, et al. Development of evidence-based recommendations for procedure-specific pain management: PROSPECT methodology. Anaesthesia 2019;74:1298–304.
31. Thybo KH, Hagi-Pedersen D, Dahl JB, et al. Effect of combination of paracetamol (acetaminophen) and ibuprofen vs either alone on patient-controlled morphine consumption in the first 24 hours after total hip arthroplasty: the PANSAID Randomized Clinical Trial. JAMA 2019;321:562–71.

32. Candido KD, Perozo OJ, Knezevic NN. Pharmacology of acetaminophen, nonsteroidal antiinflammatory drugs, and steroid medications: implications for anesthesia or unique associated risks. Anesthesiol Clin 2017;35:e145–62.

33. Marret E, Kurdi O, Zufferey P, et al. Effects of nonsteroidal antiinflammatory drugs on patient-controlled analgesia morphine side effects: meta-analysis of randomized controlled trials. Anesthesiology 2005;102:1249–60.

34. Fillingham YA, Hannon CP, Roberts KC, et al. The efficacy and safety of nonsteroidal anti-inflammatory drugs in total joint arthroplasty: systematic review and direct meta-analysis. J Arthroplasty 2020;35:2739–58.

35. Hsu JR, Mir H, Wally MK, et al. Orthopaedic trauma association musculoskeletal pain task F. clinical practice guidelines for pain management in acute musculoskeletal injury. J Orthop Trauma 2019;33:e158–82.

36. Gan TJ, Belani KG, Bergese S, et al. Fourth consensus guidelines for the management of postoperative nausea and vomiting. Anesth Analg 2020;131:411–48.

37. Rhen T, Cidlowski JA. Antiinflammatory action of glucocorticoids–new mechanisms for old drugs. N Engl J Med 2005;353:1711–23.

38. Sharma M, Gupta S, Purohit S, et al. The effect of intravenous dexamethasone on intraoperative and early postoperative pain in lumbar spine surgery: a randomized double-blind placebo-controlled study. Anesth Essays Res 2018;12:803–8.

39. De Oliveira GS Jr, Almeida MD, Benzon HT, et al. Perioperative single dose systemic dexamethasone for postoperative pain: a meta-analysis of randomized controlled trials. Anesthesiology 2011;115:575–88.

40. Waldron NH, Jones CA, Gan TJ, et al. Impact of perioperative dexamethasone on postoperative analgesia and side-effects: systematic review and meta-analysis. Br J Anaesth 2013;110:191–200.

41. Heesen M, Rijs K, Hilber N, et al. Effect of intravenous dexamethasone on postoperative pain after spinal anaesthesia - a systematic review with meta-analysis and trial sequential analysis. Anaesthesia 2019;74:1047–56.

42. Herbst RA, Telford OT, Hunting J, et al. The effects of perioperative dexamethasone on glycemic control and postoperative outcomes. Endocr Pract 2020;26:218–25.

43. Tiippana EM, Hamunen K, Kontinen VK, et al. Do surgical patients benefit from perioperative gabapentin/pregabalin? A systematic review of efficacy and safety. Anesth Analg 2007;104:1545–56.

44. Doleman B, Heinink TP, Read DJ, et al. A systematic review and meta-regression analysis of prophylactic gabapentin for postoperative pain. Anaesthesia 2015;70:1186–204.

45. Arumugam S, Lau CS, Chamberlain RS. Use of preoperative gabapentin significantly reduces postoperative opioid consumption: a meta-analysis. J Pain Res 2016;9:631–40.

46. Savelloni J, Gunter H, Lee KC, et al. Risk of respiratory depression with opioids and concomitant gabapentinoids. J Pain Res 2017;10:2635–41.

47. Fabritius ML, Geisler A, Petersen PL, et al. Gabapentin for post-operative pain management - a systematic review with meta-analyses and trial sequential analyses. Acta Anaesthesiol Scand 2016;60:1188–208.

48. Kharasch ED, Clark JD, Kheterpal S. Perioperative gabapentinoids: deflating the bubble. Anesthesiology 2020;133:251–4.

49. Hah J, Mackey SC, Schmidt P, et al. Effect of perioperative gabapentin on postoperative pain resolution and opioid cessation in a mixed surgical cohort: a randomized clinical trial. JAMA Surg 2018;153:303–11.

50. Woolf CJ, Thompson SW. The induction and maintenance of central sensitization is dependent on N-methyl-D-aspartic acid receptor activation; implications for the treatment of post-injury pain hypersensitivity states. Pain 1991;44:293–9.

51. Mion G, Villevieille T. Ketamine pharmacology: an update (pharmacodynamics and molecular aspects, recent findings). CNS Neurosci Ther 2013;19:370–80.

52. Schwenk ES, Viscusi ER, Buvanendran A, et al. Consensus Guidelines on the Use of Intravenous Ketamine Infusions for Acute Pain Management From the American Society of Regional Anesthesia and Pain Medicine, the American Academy of Pain Medicine, and the American Society of Anesthesiologists. Reg Anesth Pain Med 2018;43:456–66.

53. Zeballos JL, Lirk P, Rathmell JP. Low-Dose Ketamine for Acute Pain Management: A Timely Nudge Toward Multimodal Analgesia. Reg Anesth Pain Med 2018;43:453–5.

54. Laskowski K, Stirling A, McKay WP, et al. A systematic review of intravenous ketamine for postoperative analgesia. Can J Anaesth 2011;58:911–23.

55. Loftus RW, Yeager MP, Clark JA, et al. Intraoperative ketamine reduces perioperative opiate consumption in opiate-dependent patients with chronic back pain undergoing back surgery. Anesthesiology 2010;113:639–46.

56. Boenigk K, Echevarria GC, Nisimov E, et al. Low-dose ketamine infusion reduces postoperative hydromorphone requirements in opioid-tolerant patients following spinal fusion: a randomised controlled trial. Eur J Anaesthesiol 2019;36:8–15.

57. Sharma S, Balireddy RK, Vorenkamp KE, et al. Beyond opioid patient-controlled analgesia: a systematic review of analgesia after major spine surgery. Reg Anesth Pain Med 2012;37:79–98.

58. Avidan MS, Maybrier HR, Abdallah AB, et al. Intraoperative ketamine for prevention of postoperative delirium or pain after major surgery in older adults: an international, multicentre, double-blind, randomised clinical trial. Lancet 2017;390:267–75.

59. McNicol ED, Schumann R, Haroutounian S. A systematic review and meta-analysis of ketamine for the prevention of persistent post-surgical pain. Acta Anaesthesiol Scand 2014;58:1199–213.

60. Tramer MR, Schneider J, Marti RA, et al. Role of magnesium sulfate in postoperative analgesia. Anesthesiology 1996;84:340–7.

61. De Oliveira GS Jr, Castro-Alves LJ, Khan JH, et al. Perioperative systemic magnesium to minimize postoperative pain: a meta-analysis of randomized controlled trials. Anesthesiology 2013;119:178–90.

62. Albrecht E, Kirkham KR, Liu SS, et al. Peri-operative intravenous administration of magnesium sulphate and postoperative pain: a meta-analysis. Anaesthesia 2013;68:79–90.

63. Murphy JD, Paskaradevan J, Eisler LL, et al. Analgesic efficacy of continuous intravenous magnesium infusion as an adjuvant to morphine for postoperative analgesia: a systematic review and meta-analysis. Middle East J Anaesthesiol 2013;22:11–20.

64. Guo BL, Lin Y, Hu W, et al. Effects of Systemic Magnesium on Post-operative Analgesia: Is the Current Evidence Strong Enough? Pain Physician 2015;18:405–18.

65. Rodriguez-Rubio L, Nava E, Del Pozo JSG, et al. Influence of the perioperative administration of magnesium sulfate on the total dose of anesthetics during general anesthesia. A systematic review and meta-analysis. J Clin Anesth 2017;39:129–38.

66. Bujalska-Zadrozny M, Tatarkiewicz J, Kulik K, et al. Magnesium enhances opioid-induced analgesia - what we have learnt in the past decades? Eur J Pharm Sci 2017;99:113-27.

67. Blaudszun G, Lysakowski C, Elia N, et al. Effect of perioperative systemic alpha2 agonists on postoperative morphine consumption and pain intensity: systematic review and meta-analysis of randomized controlled trials. Anesthesiology 2012; 116:1312-22.

68. Nguyen V, Tiemann D, Park E, et al. Alpha-2 Agonists. Anesthesiol Clin 2017;35: 233-45.

69. Devereaux PJ, Sessler DI, Leslie K, et al. Clonidine in patients undergoing noncardiac surgery. N Engl J Med 2014;370:1504-13.

70. Ungur AL, Neumann T, Borchers F, et al. Perioperative management of alcohol withdrawal syndrome. Visc Med 2020;36:160-6.

71. Hidalgo MP, Auzani JA, Rumpel LC, et al. The clinical effect of small oral clonidine doses on perioperative outcomes in patients undergoing abdominal hysterectomy. Anesth Analg 2005;100:795-802.

72. Lewis SR, Nicholson A, Smith AF, et al. Alpha-2 adrenergic agonists for the prevention of shivering following general anaesthesia. Cochrane Database Syst Rev 2015;8:CD011107.

73. Schnabel A, Meyer-Friessem CH, Reichl SU, et al. Is intraoperative dexmedetomidine a new option for postoperative pain treatment? A meta-analysis of randomized controlled trials. Pain 2013;154:1140-9.

74. Le Bot A, Michelet D, Hilly J, et al. Efficacy of intraoperative dexmedetomidine compared with placebo for surgery in adults: a meta-analysis of published studies. Minerva Anestesiol 2015;81:1105-17.

75. Liu Y, Liang F, Liu X, et al. Dexmedetomidine Reduces Perioperative Opioid Consumption and Postoperative Pain Intensity in Neurosurgery: A Meta-analysis. J Neurosurg Anesthesiol 2018;30:146-55.

76. Tsaousi GG, Pourzitaki C, Aloisio S, et al. Dexmedetomidine as a sedative and analgesic adjuvant in spine surgery: a systematic review and meta-analysis of randomized controlled trials. Eur J Clin Pharmacol 2018;74:1377-89.

77. Singh PM, Panwar R, Borle A, et al. Perioperative analgesic profile of dexmedetomidine infusions in morbidly obese undergoing bariatric surgery: a meta-analysis and trial sequential analysis. Surg Obes Relat Dis 2017;13:1434-46.

78. Calderon P, Deltenre P, Stany I, et al. Clonidine administration during intraoperative monitoring for pediatric scoliosis surgery: Effects on central and peripheral motor responses. Neurophysiol Clin 2018;48:93-102.

79. Kaye AD, Chernobylsky DJ, Thakur P, et al. Dexmedetomidine in enhanced recovery after surgery (ERAS) protocols for postoperative pain. Curr Pain Headache Rep 2020;24:21.

80. Kerr DR, Kohan L. Local infiltration analgesia: a technique for the control of acute postoperative pain following knee and hip surgery: a case study of 325 patients. Acta Orthop 2008;79:174-83.

81. Zhao Y, Huang Z, Ma W. Comparison of adductor canal block with local infiltration analgesia in primary total knee arthroplasty: a meta-analysis of randomized controlled trials. Int J Surg 2019;69:89-97.

82. Anger M, Valovska T, Beloeil H, et al. PROSPECT guideline for total hip arthroplasty: a systematic review and procedure-specific postoperative pain management recommendations. Anaesthesia 2021;76:1082-97.

83. Li JW, Ma YS, Xiao LK. Postoperative Pain Management in Total Knee Arthroplasty. Orthop Surg 2019;11:755-61.

84. Andersen LO, Kehlet H. Analgesic efficacy of local infiltration analgesia in hip and knee arthroplasty: a systematic review. Br J Anaesth 2014;113:360–74.

85. Terkawi AS, Mavridis D, Sessler DI, et al. Pain management modalities after total knee arthroplasty: a network meta-analysis of 170 randomized controlled trials. Anesthesiology 2017;126:923–37.

86. Ilfeld BM, Duke KB, Donohue MC. The association between lower extremity continuous peripheral nerve blocks and patient falls after knee and hip arthroplasty. Anesth Analg 2010;111:1552–4.

87. Jaeger P, Koscielniak-Nielsen ZJ, Hilsted KL, et al. Adductor Canal Block With 10 mL Versus 30 mL Local Anesthetics and Quadriceps Strength: A Paired, Blinded, Randomized Study in Healthy Volunteers. Reg Anesth Pain Med 2015; 40:553–8.

88. Jaeger P, Nielsen ZJ, Henningsen MH, et al. Adductor canal block versus femoral nerve block and quadriceps strength: a randomized, double-blind, placebo-controlled, crossover study in healthy volunteers. Anesthesiology 2013;118: 409–15.

89. Jaeger P, Zaric D, Fomsgaard JS, et al. Adductor canal block versus femoral nerve block for analgesia after total knee arthroplasty: a randomized, double-blind study. Reg Anesth Pain Med 2013;38:526–32.

90. Chen J, Zhou C, Ma C, et al. Which is the best analgesia treatment for total knee arthroplasty: Adductor canal block, periarticular infiltration, or liposomal bupivacaine? A network meta-analysis. J Clin Anesth 2021;68:110098.

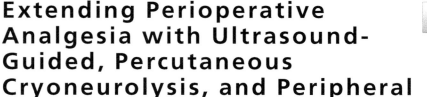

Extending Perioperative Analgesia with Ultrasound-Guided, Percutaneous Cryoneurolysis, and Peripheral Nerve Stimulation (Neuromodulation)

Rodney A. Gabriel, MD, MAS[a], Brian M. Ilfeld, MD, MS[a,b],*

KEYWORDS

- Cryoneurolysis • Neuromodulation • Ultrasound • Analgesia
- Peripheral nerve stimulation

KEY POINTS

- Ultrasound-guided percutaneous cryoneurolysis of peripheral nerves is a potential modality for management of perioperative pain that may provide months of analgesia with just a single application.
- Ultrasound-guided percutaneous neuromodulation of peripheral nerves is a potential modality for management of perioperative pain that may provide months of analgesia while also avoiding sensory and motor blockade.
- More high-quality prospective trials are needed and are underway to demonstrate their efficacy.

INTRODUCTION

Multimodal analgesia regimens are an important component in the management of acute surgical pain. Key to a successful approach to improving postoperative analgesia and reducing opioid requirements is the use of regional anesthesia, which has traditionally required local anesthetic—either a single injection or perineural catheter—administered either around peripheral nerves or within a fascial plane.

[a] Division of Regional Anesthesia and Acute Pain medicine, Department of Anesthesiology, University of California, San Diego, 200 West Arbor Drive, San Diego, California 92103-8990, USA; [b] Department of Anesthesiology, 9500 Gilman Drive, MC 0898, La Jolla, CA 92093-0898, USA
* Corresponding author. Department of Anesthesiology, 9500 Gilman Drive, MC 0898, La Jolla, CA 92093-0898.
E-mail address: bilfeld@health.ucsd.edu

Anesthesiology Clin 40 (2022) 469–479
https://doi.org/10.1016/j.anclin.2022.05.002
1932-2275/22/© 2022 Elsevier Inc. All rights reserved.
anesthesiology.theclinics.com

Unfortunately, the realistic duration even with ambulatory continuous peripheral nerve blocks usually does not match the duration of surgical pain, comprising a major limitation. Additional limitations include the risk of infection,[1] catheter dislodgement, patient burden carrying a local anesthetic reservoir and infusion pump, and rapid reservoir exhaustion.[2]

Inadequately controlled acute pain in the period after surgery is one of the greatest risk factors for the development of chronic pain.[3] One prospective study found that higher acute postoperative pain nearly tripled the odds of developing moderate-to-severe chronic pain.[4] It therefore follows that improving postoperative analgesia could greatly decrease the incidence of persistent postmastectomy pain with associated decrease in physical and mental health.[5] Indeed, single-injection peripheral nerve blocks lasting less than 1 day have decreased persistent postmastectomy pain at 3 and 12 months.[6,7] Extending the peripheral nerve block 2 days with a perineural local anesthetic infusion further decreased the incidence of chronic pain.[8] By providing potent analgesia for 2 to 3 months—essentially outlasting the pain of the surgery—chronic pain may theoretically be averted.

In this review, the use of 2 interventional modalities—ultrasound-guided percutaneous cryoneurolysis and peripheral nerve stimulation—that provide 2 to 3 months of analgesia is discussed, both of which may be used to treat acute and subacute pain and may therefore have a positive impact on the incidence and severity of chronic pain development.

CRYONEUROLYSIS

Cryoneurolysis involves the freezing of peripheral nerves to temperatures that destroy the myelin sheath and thus reduce nerve conduction, which, in turn, decreases pain signaling. The pain relief associated with cryoneurolysis may also be termed "cryoanalgesia." This should be contrasted to "cryoablation," which involves temperatures much lower that cryoneurolysis and leads to permanent tissue loss. With temperatures of cryoneurolysis between $-20°C$ and $-100°C$, Wallerian degeneration occurs distal to the lesion, which then inhibits afferent and efferent signal transmission.[9] As long as the temperature remains warmer than $-100°C$, the endoneurium, perineurium, and epineurium remain intact.[10] Because these neural layers are preserved, regeneration occurs at about 1 to 2 mm/d from the point of treatment distally, leading to full motor and sensory recovery over time.[11] In a mixed somatosensory nerve, neither the motor nor the sensory component is spared with cryoneurolysis, which is important to consider when deciding if cryoneurolysis would be clinically appropriate.[12]

Until recently, perioperative cryoneurolysis has been applied almost exclusively by surgeons directly to peripheral nerves through surgical incision. With the rapid development of ultrasound-guided regional anesthesia over the past decade, perioperative percutaneous cryoneurolysis has become more viable.[12] This modality involves the introduction of a cryoneurolysis probe inserted percutaneously and placed adjacent to the target nerve under ultrasound guidance. Once the probe tip is in an appropriate position, the operator can initiate the cryo process. Modern cryoprobes consist of a hollow tube with a smaller inner tube (**Fig. 1**). The highly pressurized gas travels from the proximal component of the inner tube to the distal end where it travels through a narrow annulus; here gas rapidly expands within the closed tip.[12] The drop in pressure is accompanied by a drop in temperature due to the Joule-Thomson effect, creating an ice ball at the tip of the probe. The cold gas does not enter the patient's tissue and is instead vented back proximally through the outer compartment. Cryoneurolysis uses a gas source to produce the extremely cold temperatures,

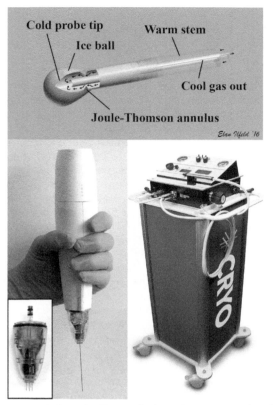

Fig. 1. A modern cryoneurolysis probe ("cannula") produces extremely cold temperatures at its tip due to the Joule-Thomson effect resulting from gas flowing from a high- to low-pressure chamber. Examples of handheld (*left panel*; Iovera Focused Cold Therapy, Myoscience, Fremont, CA, USA, with inset of optional trident probe) and portable console (*right panel*; PainBlocker, Epimed International, Inc, Farmers Branch, TX, USA) cryoneurolytic devices. (Used with permission from Brian M. Ilfeld, MD, MS.)

either with nitrous oxide or with carbon dioxide. The boiling points of the former and latter gases are −88°C and −78°C, respectively, and thus treatment of nerves with cryoneurolysis will remain at ranges that spare the endoneurium, perineurium, and epineurium.[13] Several cycles can be performed during treatment, which includes a period—usually 1 to 2 minutes—for freezing and a period for thawing—usually 30 to 60 seconds. More than 1 cycle is frequently used, although the optimal duration and number of cycles remains unexamined and unknown. There have been several case reports, case series, and observational studies describing its use in acute surgical pain management, yet few randomized controlled studies.[14,15]

Clinical Application of Percutaneous Cryoneurolysis

Dasa and colleagues[16] used a blind approach to block the anterior femoral cutaneous nerve and the infrapatellar branch of the saphenous nerve for management of postoperative pain after total knee arthroplasty. In this randomized, double-masked, sham-controlled pilot study, the use of cryoneurolysis reduced opioid consumption up to 12 weeks following surgery. Although published only in abstract form and never in the peer-reviewed literature, this investigation, nevertheless, suggested the promise of long-term benefits far outlasting the treatment itself.

Subsequently, a similar trial was published in the peer-reviewed literature. In an unmasked clinical trial, patients undergoing total knee arthroplasty randomly received preoperative percutaneous cryoneurolysis of the anterior femoral cutaneous nerve and the infrapatellar branch of the saphenous nerve or no cryo procedure.[14] The prospectively defined statistical plan specified an intention-to-treat analysis with average daily opioid consumption over the first 6 weeks as the primary outcome measure. Participants who had received cryoneurolysis (n = 62) consumed 4.8 mg/d versus 6.1 mg/d for the control group (n = 62, P = .084). However, after excluding patients with medication deviations or missing follow-up data—a "per protocol" analysis—these results were 4.2 versus 5.9 mg/d (P = .019). Because the primary outcome was negative using the intention-to-treat analysis, the secondary outcomes were not considered positive regardless of the P values for each comparison. Therefore, the results should be considered as pilot data requiring confirmation with a subsequent trial. However, the results are promising, with the treatment group consuming less opioid through the 12th week and reporting lower pain scores through the 6th week (with the per-protocol analysis; intention-to-treat results were not provided). Unfortunately, differences between treatments were minimal for range of motion and the up-and-go test but treated participants did show improvement in the Knee Injury and Osteoarthritis Outcome Score for Joint Replacement (KOOS JR) through the 12th week (P < .0001).

Multiple case reports/series described the use of ultrasound-guided percutaneous cryoneurolysis for acute pain management in surgical patients.[17–23] These included reports on applying cryoneurolysis to the infrapatellar branch preoperatively for patients undergoing total knee arthroplasty,[19] suprascapular nerve for patients undergoing rotator cuff repair,[19] intercostal nerves to treat refractory pain following nephrolithotomy,[17] subcostal and intercostal nerves preoperatively or in patients undergoing iliac crest bone grafting,[17] sciatic and femoral nerve in patients who underwent lower limb amputation,[23] lateral femoral cutaneous nerves for patients who underwent skin grafting for burn surgery,[20] intercostal nerves for patients following traumatic rib fractures,[18] intercostal nerves preoperatively in patients undergoing mastectomy,[21] and intercostal nerves after severe chest trauma.[24] In the case series consisting of 3 patients receiving cryoneurolysis at multiple intercostal levels before mastectomy, the mean pain score on the numeric rating scale over multiple postoperative days (up to postoperative day 28) was 0 and none used supplemental opioids during this period.[21]

In a randomized, double-masked, sham-controlled pilot study, patients with burns (n = 12) undergoing split-thickness skin graft harvesting received a lateral femoral cutaneous nerve block followed by either sham or active ultrasound-guided percutaneous cryoneurolysis.[15] Subjects randomized to the active group reported lower average and maximum pain scores (up to postoperative day 21), required less opioids (up to postoperative day 21), and reported fewer sleep disturbances (up to postoperative day 2).

Specific contraindications to cryoneurolysis include cold urticaria, Raynaud disease, cryoglobulinemia, and paroxysmal cold hemoglobinuria.[12] There are few large studies available that may be used to estimate the incidence of complications; however, fortunately, the available literature is overwhelmingly positive.[12] Before the introduction of ultrasound-guided percutaneous cryoneurolysis, most reports for acute pain involved intraoperative application during thoracotomy.[25–33] Two of these randomized controlled trials reported an increase in neuropathic pain associated with use of intraoperative cryoneurolysis when administered via surgical incision.[27,31]

However, far more failed to find any increase in neuropathic pain. The reason for the differing findings may be the variable techniques used by the many investigators. Some surgeons describe dissecting down to the nerve, lifting it out of its surrounding tissue with an instrument or suture, and then applying the cryo probe directly to the nerve—often in 2 different locations. The combination of applying cryoneurolysis and nerve retraction from the surgical incision may contribute to a "double crush" phenomenon, which potentially may have increased the incidence of subsequent neuropathic pain. When investigators attempted to induce chronic pain in rats with cryoneurolysis, they could only do so if they manipulated the nerve during the procedure—if the nerve was left undisturbed during the cryo treatment, chronic pain was never observed.[9] These preclinical results suggest that percutaneous application of cryoneurolysis should not have a similar risk of neuropathy; and, indeed, no reports of increased chronic pain have been published to date using the percutaneous technique.

Percutaneous cryoneurolysis—either via ultrasound guidance or landmark techniques—is a US Food and Drug Administration (FDA)-cleared alternative to continuous peripheral nerve blocks for some indications. Percutaneous cryoneurolysis is especially appropriate when long-term blockade of sensory nerves is desired for procedures leading to postoperative pain that may extend passed the duration of traditional local anesthetic nerve blocks. Because a single cryoneurolysis application has the potential to last several months, cryoneurolysis has fewer applicable surgical procedures than shorter-duration local anesthetic-based blocks. However, when applied appropriately, percutaneous cryoneurolysis has the potential to provide ultra-long-duration analgesia with a single preoperative treatment requiring no subsequent management and external equipment and without the risk of toxicity. Adequately powered randomized controlled trials are needed to validate the technique in the multitude of possible applications, quantify its efficacy, and estimate its risks.

PERCUTANEOUS PERIPHERAL NERVE STIMULATION (NEUROMODULATION)

Neuromodulation involves the use of electrical stimulation to provide analgesia. The mechanism of action of this modality has yet to be explained definitively, but the primary mechanism is believed to be related to the concept of "gate control" theory, in which stimulation of large-diameter afferent fibers inhibits the transmission of pain signals from small-diameter pain fibers to the central nervous system at the level of the spinal cord.[34,35] The use of peripheral neuromodulation is not new in chronic pain management.[36] However, more recently developed technology allowing a less invasive percutaneous approach using ultrasound has enabled application to acute pain such as postoperative pain.[37] The technique involves percutaneously inserting an electric lead under ultrasound guidance in proximity to a target nerve. A pulse generator ("stimulator") may be temporarily affixed on the surface of the skin (**Fig. 2**). This process contrasts with surgically placing leads with an implanted stimulator, which is far more invasive and may require a dedicated procedure suite/operating room. In contrast, ultrasound-guided percutaneous lead insertion may be achieved in the same setting in which a catheter-based regional anesthesia technique is placed (eg, preoperative block area).

Percutaneous peripheral nerve stimulation has potential advantages over perineural catheters placed for continuous infusions. Sensory, proprioception, and motor nerves are spared, a characteristic that is both beneficial and unique in regional anesthesia. The single US FDA-cleared lead has an extraordinarily low rate of infection (1 infection in more than 32,000 indwelling days).[38] This low risk of infection is theoretically due to

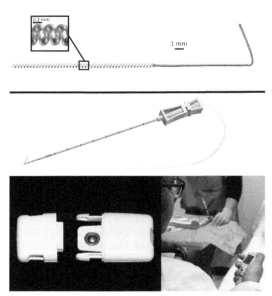

Fig. 2. A percutaneous peripheral nerve stimulation system approved by the US Food and Drug Administration to treat acute pain (OnePass, SPR Therapeutics, Cleveland, OH, USA). The insulated lead (MicroLead, SPR Therapeutics) is 0.2 mm in diameter wrapped into a helical coil 0.6 mm in diameter (*top panel*), which is percutaneously inserted using a preloaded introducer (*middle panel*). The rechargeable battery snaps into the pulse generator (SPRINT PNS System, SPR Therapeutics) and is controlled with a handheld remote control (*bottom panels*). (Used with permission from Brian M. Ilfeld, MD, MS.)

the helical coil design, which allows fibrosis between coils that creates a seal blocking passage of superficial pathogens and stops transdermal "pistoning" observed with cylindrical perineural catheters. There is a lower patient burden with no infusion pump or local anesthetic reservoir to carry. Sleep is not disturbed by noise as caused by an electronic infusion pump, and there is no risk of anesthetic leakage or toxicity. The risk of dislodgement seems to be lower than for perineural catheters, possibly due to the helically coiled lead that will extend by partially unraveling like a spring without pulling out the end. Last, the leads are approved to remain in situ for a much longer period compared with local anesthetic-based perineural catheters, with the currently FDA-cleared lead approved for up to 60 indwelling days.[39]

Disadvantages include a greater insertion time requirement than for perineural catheters, a complete lack of a surgical block, lower analgesic potency than a single-injection nerve block, lead fracture (although no negative sequelae have been reported), lead removal requiring a health care provider (catheters can be withdrawn at home by the patients themselves), and the cost of the device, which is currently many multiples of a perineural local anesthetic infusion. Importantly, far more patient understanding and cooperation is required to adequately apply neuromodulation relative to perineural local anesthetic infusion.

Clinical Applications of Percutaneous Peripheral Neuromodulation

Initial proof-of-concept reports of percutaneous peripheral nerve stimulation to treat acute pain involved small series of patients who had total knee arthroplasty and residual pain resistant to opioids.[40–42] Subsequently, small feasibility studies described neuromodulation to treat postoperative pain for up to 1 month following total knee arthroplasty,[43] hallux valgus repair,[44] rotator cuff repair,[45] and anterior cruciate ligament repair.[46] In the 3 latter studies, patients received preoperative lead insertion and underwent 3 stages of treatment in the recovery room: (1) active or sham activation for 5 minutes determined randomly, (2) crossover treatment for another 5 minutes, and (3) 30 additional minutes of active stimulation. Subsequently, active stimulation was continued for 2 to 4 weeks. Decreases in pain were observed during active stimulation, and longer-term follow-up suggested remarkably low opioid consumption and pain scores beginning the day following surgery (many participants required a single-injection peripheral nerve block in the recovery room to achieve discharge criteria).

Finally, there is a single published multicenter, randomized, double-masked, sham-controlled pilot study completed to help plan for a subsequent definitive trial (n = 66).[47] Preoperatively, electrical leads were percutaneously implanted using ultrasound to target the sciatic nerve for major foot/ankle surgery, femoral nerve for anterior cruciate ligament reconstruction, and the brachial plexus for rotator cuff repair. Participants were discharged home with either an active or sham pulse generator and had their leads removed during their 2-week postoperative surgical appointment. The dual primary outcome measures were both positive. The average pain scores over the first postoperative week measured using a 0 to 10 Numeric Rating Scale for subjects receiving active stimulation was a mean of 1.1 versus 3.1 for participants receiving sham ($P < .001$). The cumulative opioid consumption for the first postoperative week for participants receiving active stimulation was 5 mg versus 48 mg for subjects receiving sham ($P < .001$). These treatment effects were far larger than anticipated, with pain scores reduced by 65% and opioid consumption reduced by 90%. Secondary outcomes revealed reduced average and maximum daily pain scores and opioid consumption on postoperative days 1 to 4, 7, and 11. The lower pain levels translated into far less interference of pain in daily physical and emotional functioning as measured by the interference subscale of the Brief Pain Inventory. On subgroup analysis separating participants who had brachial plexus or sciatic nerve leads/stimulation, both cohorts demonstrated similar benefits in opioid consumption and pain scores.[48] Completion of the definitive multicenter, randomized, controlled trial is anticipated in 2023 (clinicaltrials.gov NCT04713098).

SUMMARY

Ultrasound-guided percutaneous cryoneurolysis and peripheral nerve stimulation are relatively unique options with somewhat distinctive potential benefits treating acute pain. Their relative benefits differentiate them from each other: cryoneurolysis may be applied to many nerves, whereas a neuromodulation lead will impact only 1 nerve or plexus (although multiple leads may be used simultaneously). Cryoneurolysis requires no patient assistance, whereas neuromodulation requires the highest level of patient understanding and assistance to optimize both lead insertion and subsequent pulse generator management. Relatedly, cryoneurolysis has no equipment that can fail or leads that may dislodge/fracture unlike neuromodulation. And although cryoneurolysis has the up-front cost of the device, per-patient costs are relatively negligible. In contrast, neuromodulation has no up-front costs but relatively high per-patient costs.

Percutaneous peripheral nerve stimulation allows for analgesia titration, whereas cryoneurolysis does not; also, neuromodulation induces no motor, sensory, or proprioception deficits, unlike cryoneurolysis. Neuromodulation leads may be removed at any time, whereas the duration of cryoneurolysis cannot be purposefully truncated following application and is highly variable and unpredictable. What both techniques offer is the possibility of providing analgesia that outlasts the pain from the initial surgical procedure, thereby dramatically improving both acute pain and possibly the incidence and severity of chronic pain, all with surprisingly few risks identified to date. However, only with persistent, unbiased investigation will the true benefits and risks of these 2 modalities be realized (NCT03286543, NCT04713098, NCT04341948, NCT04198662, NCT03578237).[49]

CLINICS CARE POINTS

- When deciding an optimal canddiate for ultrasound-guided percutaneous cryoanalgesia, the provider must weigh the risk and benefits of analgesia to that of prolonged motor and sensory blockade.
- When deciding an optimal candidate for percutaneous peripheral neuromodulation for patients undergoing surgery, the provider must also assess the patients' buy-in and ability to cooperate with the postoperative management of the device system

REFERENCES

1. Capdevila X, Bringuier S, Borgeat A. Infectious risk of continuous peripheral nerve blocks. Anesthesiology 2009;110:182–8.
2. Ilfeld BM. Continuous peripheral nerve blocks: an update of the published evidence and comparison with novel, alternative analgesic modalities. Anesth Analg 2017;124:308–35.
3. Kehlet H, Jensen TS, Woolf CJ. Persistent postsurgical pain: risk factors and prevention. Lancet 2006;367:1618–25.
4. Andersen KG, Duriaud HM, Jensen HE, et al. Predictive factors for the development of persistent pain after breast cancer surgery. Pain 2015;156:2413–22.
5. Peuckmann V, Ekholm O, Rasmussen NK, et al. Chronic pain and other sequelae in long-term breast cancer survivors: nationwide survey in Denmark. Eur J Pain 2009;13:478–85.
6. Qian B, Huang S, Liao X, et al. Serratus anterior plane block reduces the prevalence of chronic postsurgical pain after modified radical mastectomy: A randomized controlled trial. J Clin Anesth 2021;74:110410.
7. Fujii T, Shibata Y, Akane A, et al. A randomised controlled trial of pectoral nerve-2 (PECS 2) block vs. serratus plane block for chronic pain after mastectomy. Anaesthesia 2019;74:1558–62.
8. Ilfeld BM, Madison SJ, Suresh PJ, et al. Persistent postmastectomy pain and pain-related physical and emotional functioning with and without a continuous paravertebral nerve block: a prospective 1-year follow-up assessment of a randomized, triple-masked, placebo-controlled study. Ann Surg Oncol 2015;22: 2017–25.
9. Wagner R, DeLeo JA, Heckman HM, et al. Peripheral nerve pathology following sciatic cryoneurolysis: relationship to neuropathic behaviors in the rat. Exp Neurol 1995;133:256–64.
10. Zhou L, Kambin P, Casey KF, et al. Mechanism research of cryoanalgesia. Neurol Res 1995;17:307–11.

11. Shah SB, Bremner S, Esparza M, et al. Does cryoneurolysis result in persistent motor deficits? A controlled study using a rat peroneal nerve injury model. Reg Anesth Pain Med 2020;45:287–92.
12. Ilfeld BM, Finneran JJ. Cryoneurolysis and Percutaneous Peripheral Nerve Stimulation to Treat Acute Pain. Anesthesiology 2020;133:1127–49.
13. Evans PJ. Cryoanalgesia. The application of low temperatures to nerves to produce anaesthesia or analgesia. Anaesthesia 1981;36:1003–13.
14. Mihalko WM, Kerkhof AL, Ford MC, et al. Cryoneurolysis before Total Knee Arthroplasty in Patients With Severe Osteoarthritis for Reduction of Postoperative Pain and Opioid Use in a Single-Center Randomized Controlled Trial. J Arthroplasty 2021;36:1590–8.
15. Finneran Iv JJ, Schaar AN, Swisher MW, et al. Percutaneous cryoneurolysis of the lateral femoral cutaneous nerve for analgesia following skin grafting: a randomized, controlled pilot study. Reg Anesth Pain Med 2021;47(1):60–1.
16. Dasa VD, Lensing G, Parsons M, et al. An ancient treatment for present-day surgery: percutaneous freezing sensory nerves for treatment of postsurgical knee pain. Tech Reg Anesth Pain Manage 2015;18:145–9.
17. Gabriel RA, Finneran JJ, Asokan D, et al. Ultrasound-Guided percutaneous cryoneurolysis for acute pain management: a case report. A A Case Rep 2017;9:129–32.
18. Finneran Iv JJ, Gabriel RA, Swisher MW, et al. Ultrasound-guided percutaneous intercostal nerve cryoneurolysis for analgesia following traumatic rib fracture -a case series. Korean J Anesthesiol 2020;73:455–9.
19. Ilfeld BM, Gabriel RA, Trescot AM. Ultrasound-guided percutaneous cryoneurolysis providing postoperative analgesia lasting many weeks following a single administration: a replacement for continuous peripheral nerve blocks?: a case report. Korean J Anesthesiol 2017;70:567–70.
20. Finneran JJ, Swisher MW, Gabriel RA, et al. Ultrasound-Guided Lateral Femoral Cutaneous Nerve Cryoneurolysis for Analgesia in Patients With Burns. J Burn Care Res 2020;41:224–7.
21. Gabriel RA, Finneran JJ, Swisher MW, et al. Ultrasound-guided percutaneous intercostal cryoanalgesia for multiple weeks of analgesia following mastectomy: a case series. Korean J Anesthesiol 2020;73:163–8.
22. Vossler JD, Zhao FZ. Intercostal nerve cryoablation for control of traumatic rib fracture pain: a case report. Trauma Case Rep 2019;23:100229.
23. Gabriel RA, JJT F, Trescot AM, et al. Ultrasound-guided percutaneous cryoneurolysis for postoperative analgesia after limb amputation: a case series. A A Pract 2019;12:231–4.
24. Farley P, Mullen PR, Lee YL, et al. Intercostal cryoneurolysis after severe chest trauma: a brief report. Am Surg 2022;88(6):1336–7, 3134820943641.
25. Ba YF, Li XD, Zhang X, et al. Comparison of the analgesic effects of cryoanalgesia vs. parecoxib for lung cancer patients after lobectomy. Surg Today 2015;45:1250–4.
26. Keller BA, Kabagambe SK, Becker JC, et al. Intercostal nerve cryoablation versus thoracic epidural catheters for postoperative analgesia following pectus excavatum repair: Preliminary outcomes in twenty-six cryoablation patients. J Pediatr Surg 2016;51:2033–8.
27. Mustola ST, Lempinen J, Saimanen E, et al. Efficacy of thoracic epidural analgesia with or without intercostal nerve cryoanalgesia for postthoracotomy pain. Ann Thorac Surg 2011;91:869–73.

28. Sepsas E, Misthos P, Anagnostopulu M, et al. The role of intercostal cryoanalgesia in post-thoracotomy analgesia. Interact Cardiovasc Thorac Surg 2013;16:814–8.

29. Ju H, Feng Y, Yang BX, et al. Comparison of epidural analgesia and intercostal nerve cryoanalgesia for post-thoracotomy pain control. Eur J Pain 2008;12:378–84.

30. Yang MK, Cho CH, Kim YC. The effects of cryoanalgesia combined with thoracic epidural analgesia in patients undergoing thoracotomy. Anaesthesia 2004;59:1073–7.

31. Moorjani N, Zhao F, Tian Y, et al. Effects of cryoanalgesia on post-thoracotomy pain and on the structure of intercostal nerves: a human prospective randomized trial and a histological study. Eur J Cardiothorac Surg 2001;20:502–7.

32. Gwak MS, Yang M, Hahm TS, et al. Effect of cryoanalgesia combined with intravenous continuous analgesia in thoracotomy patients. J Korean Med Sci 2004;19:74–8.

33. Bucerius J, Metz S, Walther T, et al. Pain is significantly reduced by cryoablation therapy in patients with lateral minithoracotomy. Ann Thorac Surg 2000;70:1100–4.

34. Shealy CN, Mortimer JT, Reswick JB. Electrical inhibition of pain by stimulation of the dorsal columns: preliminary clinical report. Anesth Analg 1967;46:489–91.

35. Wall PD, Sweet WH. Temporary abolition of pain in man. Science 1967;155:108–9.

36. Stillings D. A survey of the history of electrical stimulation for pain to 1900. Med Instrum 1975;9:255–9.

37. Chae J, Yu D, Walker M. Percutaneous, intramuscular neuromuscular electrical stimulation for the treatment of shoulder subluxation and pain in chronic hemiplegia: a case report. Am J Phys Med Rehabil 2001;80:296–301.

38. Ilfeld BM, Gabriel RA, Saulino MF, et al. Infection rates of electrical leads used for percutaneous neurostimulation of the peripheral nervous system. Pain Pract 2017;17:753–62.

39. Ilfeld BM, Grant SA. Ultrasound-guided percutaneous peripheral nerve stimulation for postoperative analgesia: could neurostimulation replace continuous peripheral nerve blocks? Reg Anesth Pain Med 2016;41:720–2.

40. Ilfeld BM, Grant SA, Gilmore CA, et al. Neurostimulation for postsurgical analgesia: a novel system enabling ultrasound-guided percutaneous peripheral nerve stimulation. Pain Pract 2017;17:892–901.

41. Ilfeld BM, Ball ST, Cohen SP, et al. Percutaneous peripheral nerve stimulation to control postoperative pain, decrease opioid use, and accelerate functional recovery following orthopedic trauma. Mil Med 2019;184:557–64.

42. Ilfeld BM, Gilmore CA, Grant SA, et al. Ultrasound-guided percutaneous peripheral nerve stimulation for analgesia following total knee arthroplasty: a prospective feasibility study. J Orthop Surg Res 2017;12:4.

43. Ilfeld BM, Ball ST, Gabriel RA, et al. A feasibility study of percutaneous peripheral nerve stimulation for the treatment of postoperative pain following total knee arthroplasty. Neuromodulation 2019;22:653–60.

44. Ilfeld BM, Gabriel RA, Said ET, et al. Ultrasound-guided percutaneous peripheral nerve stimulation: neuromodulation of the sciatic nerve for postoperative analgesia following ambulatory foot surgery, a proof-of-concept study. Reg Anesth Pain Med 2018;43:580–9.

45. Ilfeld BM, JJT F, Gabriel RA, et al. Ultrasound-guided percutaneous peripheral nerve stimulation: neuromodulation of the suprascapular nerve and brachial

plexus for postoperative analgesia following ambulatory rotator cuff repair. A proof-of-concept study. Reg Anesth Pain Med 2019;44:310–8.

46. Ilfeld BM, Said ET, JJT F, et al. Ultrasound-guided percutaneous peripheral nerve stimulation: neuromodulation of the femoral nerve for postoperative analgesia following ambulatory anterior cruciate ligament reconstruction: a proof of concept study. Neuromodulation 2019;22:621–9.

47. Ilfeld BM, Plunkett A, Vijjeswarapu AM, et al. Percutaneous peripheral nerve stimulation (neuromodulation) for postoperative pain: a randomized, sham-controlled pilot study. Anesthesiology 2021;135:95–110.

48. Ilfeld BM, Plunkett A, Vijjeswarapu AM, et al. Percutaneous neuromodulation of the brachial plexus and sciatic nerve for the treatment of acute pain following surgery: secondary outcomes from a multicenter, randomized, controlled pilot study. Neuromodulation 2021. [epub ahead of print].

49. Ilfeld BM, Mariano ER. Evaluating clinical research and bloodletting (Seriously). Reg Anesth Pain Med 2010;35:448–9.

Unique Issues Related to Regional Anesthesia in Pediatric Orthopedics

Walid Alrayashi, MD[a],*, Joseph Cravero, MD[b],
Roland Brusseau, MD[c]

KEYWORDS

- Pediatric anesthesia • Regional anesthesia • Orthopedic anesthesia
- Continuous nerve block • Ambulatory catheter

KEY POINTS

- The most up-to-date practice guidelines conclude that there is sound evidence that regional blocks can and should preferably be performed under anesthesia or deep sedation in children of all ages. Conversely, registry data suggest that performing regional anesthesia in awake or only lightly sedated children actually carries an increased, albeit low, risk of postoperative neurologic symptoms.
- A joint effort of the European and American regional anesthesia societies (ESRA and ASRA) in 2015 found no convincing association between regional anesthesia and delayed diagnosis of compartment syndrome. It was concluded that there is no current evidence that the use of regional anesthetics increases the risk of ACS or delays its diagnosis in children.
- Patients with Baclofen pumps can safely receive neuraxial or paraneuraxial anesthetics with appropriate device interrogation and consultation with a neurosurgeon and the use of advanced imaging modalities such as ultrasound and fluoroscopy.

INTRODUCTION

As is the case with anesthesia for adults, orthopedic surgeries comprise a very significant portion of all pediatric anesthetics. While there is significant overlap in terms of the underlying pathology prompting procedures (eg, injury, malignancy, and so forth)

[a] Department of Anesthesiology, Harvard Medical School, Home Analgesia Program, Critical Care and Pain Medicine, Boston Children's Hospital, 300 Longwood Avenue, Boston, MA 02115, USA; [b] Department of Anesthesiology, Harvard Medical School, Critical Care and Pain Medicine, Boston Children's Hospital, 300 Longwood Avenue, Boston, MA 02115, USA; [c] Department of Anesthesiology, Harvard Medical School, Pediatric Regional Anesthesia Program, Critical Care and Pain Medicine, Boston Children's Hospital, 300 Longwood Avenue, Boston, MA 02115, USA
* Corresponding author.
E-mail address: walid.alrayashi@childrens.harvard.edu

Anesthesiology Clin 40 (2022) 481–489
https://doi.org/10.1016/j.anclin.2022.05.001
1932-2275/22/© 2022 Elsevier Inc. All rights reserved.
anesthesiology.theclinics.com

as well as anesthetic techniques, there are unique elements to anesthetic practice when working with a pediatric population.

Orthopedics cases in pediatrics fall into several categories. First, injuries, sports-related or other, comprise a major fraction of all pediatric orthopedic anesthetics. These can be joint injuries (shoulders, knees, hips) or fractures. Fracture surgery in children poses unique concerns as it may involve the patient's growth plate.

Other broad categories of pediatric orthopedic surgery include repair or mitigation of congenital anomalies, scoliosis (idiopathic or neurogenic), and malignancy. Pediatric orthopedic oncology is unique because many of the major malignancies such as osteosarcoma, Ewing's sarcoma, and rhabdomyosarcoma, usually present in childhood and adolescence and may involve limb sparing and other radical procedures that are not performed in adults.

Similar/dissimilar

While the anatomic locations are like those in adults, the distribution of cases in pediatric orthopedics is different. For example, shoulder surgery is less prevalent in pediatrics, but quite common among adults.[1] Similarly, joint replacement surgeries are rarely encountered in children. Rather, procedures designed to extend the lifespan of the existing joints are performed such as correction of misalignments, congenital dislocation, or suboptimal alignment.

Major surgeries such as periacetabular osteotomies and derotational osteotomies of the long bones are associated with large blood losses and hemodynamic instability.[2] However, when compared with adults, pediatric patients are generally able to better tolerate anesthetics and the commensurate physiologic perturbations, largely offsetting much of the increased complexity of such corrective procedures. Nevertheless, there are subgroups, such as neurologically compromised patients, whereby anesthetic management more closely mirrors that of the elderly patient.[3]

Growth of Regional Anesthesia

Perhaps the most impressive change in anesthesia for pediatric orthopedic patients has been the rapid expansion of regional anesthetic techniques in children.[4] In many centers, regional anesthesia for pediatric cases is just as common as that in adult surgeries.

Much of this growth has resulted from the widespread application of advanced ultrasound-guided techniques and the entry of subspecialty trained practitioners into the workforce.[5] Another reason for the swift adoption has been the cooperative development of large data registries that have demonstrated that pediatric regional anesthesia is extremely safe.[6]

The most recent data from the Pediatric Regional Anesthesia Database (PRAN) detail no permanent neurologic deficits in more than 100,000 blocks. Their data indicate that the risk of transient neurologic deficit was 2.4:10,000 (95% CI, 1.6–3.6:10,000) and was not different between peripheral and neuraxial blocks. The risk of severe local anesthetic systemic toxicity was 0.76:10,000 (95% CI, 0.3–1.6:10,000).[6]

Most of these registries or groups (ADARPEF, PRAN, APRICOT, and so forth) publish intermittent updates on the safety of regional anesthetics in pediatric patients and address known knowledge gaps to facilitate their investigation.[7] Other registries are now seeking to resolve questions of efficacy and comparative outcomes to further guide clinical practice.[8]

Plan

This article will focus largely on notable issues related to regional anesthesia in pediatrics. First, the controversy surrounding awake versus anesthetized block placement will be addressed. There will also be a discussion on the use of regional anesthetics in orthopedics cases and the risk of compartment syndrome.

We will also address the concern for regional anesthetics in the setting of an instrumented spine (eg, following spine fusion, baclofen pump placement) will be reviewed as such can have significant ramifications for patients.

Finally, this article will consider ambulatory regional catheters and their increasing use in pediatric orthopedic anesthesia. Their utilization during the COVD epidemic played a key role in facilitating procedures that would have otherwise been canceled due to the protracted hospital bed shortage.

DISCUSSION
Awake Versus Asleep Blocks

The controversy surrounding awake versus asleep blocks is an old one that persists to this day, even among pediatric anesthesiologists. "Old" is a relative term in pediatric regional anesthesia as pediatric regional anesthesia got its first real foothold following the first World Congress on Pediatric Pain in Seattle in the late 1980s.[9] Rapid, enthusiasm-driven adoption followed. It quickly became apparent that most of the blocks were performed with the child either anesthetized or deeply sedated. Some argued that the practice was associated with unnecessary risk—not just the risks related to both general and regional anesthesia, but also the patient's inability to report warning signs of potential nerve injury or signs of local anesthetic systemic toxicity.

This led influential pediatric anesthetists to publish a consensus statement supporting the practice of placing blocks on anesthetized patients, designating it as safe.[10] Later, 2 prospective, large-scale, multicenter studies from the ADARPEF (French Language Society of Pediatric Anesthesia) and PRAN (based on the prospective collection of more than 100,000 pediatric nerve blocks) reported a very low rate of complications.[6,7]

Recently updated practice guidelines published jointly by ESRA and ASRA concluded that there is sound evidence to recommend that regional blocks can and *should* preferably be performed under anesthesia or deep sedation in children of all ages. In fact, PRAN data suggested that performing regional anesthesia in awake or only lightly sedated children carry an *increased*, albeit exceedingly low, risk of postoperative neurologic symptoms.[11] Given this evidence, the case would seem to be closed concerning how to perform regional anesthesia in children.

This safety record is likely due to advances in ultrasound visualization and pressure limiting local anesthetic delivery systems have largely eliminated the risk of intraneural or intravascular injection.[12] An argument can still be made those certain types of local anesthetic toxicity signs and symptoms (LAST) may manifest more rapidly in an awake patient. However, there are numerous ways LAST can be recognized in the anesthetized patient, and the requisite cardiopulmonary resuscitation can be initiated very quickly in the OR environment.

Compartment Syndrome

This is another long-standing controversy that has played out quite differently (so far) depending on one's location relative to the Atlantic Ocean. The central question is whether regional analgesia obscures (or masks) the developing symptoms of acute compartment syndrome.[13]

Surgical acute compartment syndrome is the result of an increased pressure in a closed, largely inelastic fascial compartment, usually due to postinjury edema.[14] Whether this is due to an arteriovenous gradient in the setting of damaged tissues or cyclic ischemia and reperfusion injury is unclear. However, the net result is ongoing tissue breakdown until the pressure is resolved.[15]

Resolution of compartment pressure may be achieved by measures as simple as removing a cast; most pediatric casts are bivalved for this purpose. On the other hand, in some cases, patients may require a surgical fasciotomy. A diagnosis of compartment syndrome is usually a surgical emergency. Younger or cognitively impaired children present unique challenges in diagnosis and treatment given their inability to articulate symptoms such as pain and paresthesia. For some providers, this concern regarding prompt diagnosis results in greater hesitation about using regional anesthetics.

One recent report cited an incidence of acute compartment syndrome following pediatric trauma of 0.02%.[16] Age is an important predictor of the development of ACS; teenaged children have a higher prevalence of ACS following tibial fracture, consistent with adults. Younger children, however, tend to have a higher incidence of upper extremity ACS, with a rate of 0.6% for humeral and 0.7% for forearm fractures. A joint effort of the European and American Regional Anesthesia Societies (ESRA and ASRA) in 2015 found no convincing evidence of any correlation between regional anesthesia and delayed diagnosis of compartment syndrome.[17]

Furthermore, other studies have supported the use of low concentration local anesthetics in cases that were previously considered to be at high risk for compartment syndrome. These concentrations include bupivacaine 0.25% or ropivacaine 0.2% for single shots and 0.1%, respectively, for continuous infusions. They found that doing so did not increase the risk of developing ACS. In fact, ACS was promptly identified with even higher concentrations such as ropivacaine 0.75%.[18] Despite this data, debates continue regarding the use of regional anesthesia in children at risk of ACS, particularly in the United States.[19]

Whereas US-based surgeons and anesthesiologists continue to largely disagree about this, when confronted with the same data, their European counterparts opt for regional anesthetics much more commonly in patients at risk for ACS. These practitioners endorse a mechanistic basis for their practice as well as heightened monitoring.[16]

The mechanism of tissue injury is postulated to start from muscle ischemia which leads to acidosis, hydrogen ion activation, and the nonadapting activation of the pain receptors. This process is not effectively muted by local anesthetics.[20] Further, inflammatory markers associated with tissue injury and trauma may induce local anesthetic tachyphylaxis after the activation of the nociceptor.[21] Both mechanisms could explain why patients with evolving compartment syndrome might still present with breakthrough pain in the setting of a functional nerve block. This may result in earlier manifestations of detection and thus hasten the diagnosis. The converse argument could also be made that the simple belief that compartment syndrome might be masked by a block, could lead to increased awareness and monitoring of the patient's signs and symptoms.

Whether there is an ischemic pain pathway that would serve as an early warning sign, or that there is closer surveillance because of a block in this setting, there certainly is a good case to be made for regional anesthetics decreasing the incidence of unrecognized or severe compartment syndrome.

Regional Anesthesia and Implanted Spinal Hardware

Pediatric patients with intrathecal pumps *in situ* presenting for additional major surgery are likely afflicted by numerous comorbidities. Most commonly these are various forms of cerebral palsy (CP). Hip instability and dysplasia are among the most common and debilitating orthopedic deformities experienced by nonambulatory children with CP.[22] Hip reconstruction surgery has been demonstrated to improve health-related quality of life in children with CP. However, managing acute pain after this surgery can be challenging.[23] It has been shown to be more painful than posterior spine fusion surgery, emphasizing the importance of establishing safe and effective analgesic strategies in this vulnerable population.[24]

Reliable pain control for these patients is of paramount importance as these patients frequently cannot communicate their pain states. Additionally, a vicious circle develops whereby inadequate pain control leads to increased postoperative spasticity, which further worsens pain.[25] Many of these patients have intrathecal pumps delivering medications such as baclofen to reduce spasticity and these, if used in the perioperative period, can help manage this spasticity.[26] However, these pumps are often considered a contraindication to regional anesthetics, especially neuraxial approaches.

Unfortunately, this patient population is susceptible to numerous issues during their perioperative period. There is often a lack of communication between various clinical services, inadequate understanding of the patient's pain, and various unsupported beliefs about contraindications to regional anesthesia. Often these patients end up medicated with opioids leading to the expected respiratory and gastrointestinal side effects—all of which can lead to adverse outcomes in this population.[27] Recognizing this gap in effective pain management, one institution offered epidural or peripheral nerve blocks after careful multidisciplinary planning involving the anesthesiology, orthopedic, pain medicine, and neurosurgery teams. The neurosurgeons were able to interrogate the implanted device and provide guidance on the pump position, catheter track, and subarachnoid entry site. Patients were either offered epidural anesthesia primarily or regional anesthesia (eg, lumbar plexus blocks) if the former was not feasible.[28] Fluoroscopy was used to visualize the implanted materials and facilitate safe and successful placement of epidural catheters. Patients who were not good candidates for epidurals received a peripheral nerve block using ultrasound guidance. That particular study included a total cohort of 44 patients with baclofen pumps who were treated without significant complications.[29]

Exploring these techniques can offer very effective analgesia in this patient population who are at high risk for complications from solely opiate-based pain control.[30] This experience has led to a change in practice at one institution, such that all patients now receive some form of image-guided regional analgesia.[31]

Sports Medicine and Ambulatory Catheters

Sports-related injuries in young athletes continue to increase in prevalence with nearly 3 million children injured every year.[32] At the same time, opioid misuse continues to be a major issue in this vulnerable population with over 20% of senior high school students reporting misuse of prescription drugs for nonmedical purposes.[33] One claims-based cohort study of 2.7 million adolescents and young adults without cancer, demonstrated that daily opioid dosage and use were associated with increased overdose risk. In fact, in 2016, of approximately 3000 opioid-related deaths in adolescents, a third were from prescription drugs. Despite this epidemic, patients are still overprescribed opioid medications after their surgeries.[34]

One strategy currently used to reduce the need for perioperative opioids is the use of continuous nerve block techniques using indwelling catheters. These catheters can then be connected to portable pumps that allow patients to use them at home.[35] There are primarily 2 types of pumps: elastomeric and electronic. Both have pros and cons.

Elastomeric pumps are easy to set up with only one dial to set the rate, are completely mechanic with no electronic parts, are easier to transport and store, and they do not have any alarms or buttons for the patients to manage. However, they do not display the volume remaining and are limited in the volumes that can be stored in the device.[35] Alternatively, electronic pumps can be attached to any size bag, tend to be more accurate in their delivery, and will often times display the remaining volume. Downsides of these pumps include the fact that they are a little more complicated to set up, have alarms and buttons that require greater education for patients to operate, and are usually more expensive. They also rely on battery life and require extra workflow processes for patients such as the need to ship them back to the vendors or hospitals whereby they are dispensed, even though there are disposable pumps on the market.[36]

The use of these devices and techniques is still in the early adoption period compared with adult centers which have been using them for a couple of decades with great success. For example, one study that cataloged the practices in 32 Canadian hospitals, only about 6% of the pediatric centers had an organized pain service, with only half of that providing patients with ambulatory catheters.[37] This was dramatically different from adult centers whereby this was more commonplace. There are several potential reasons for the delayed application. One is related to the concern around appropriate dosing in smaller children. There is also some trepidation about monitoring children who may or may not be able to adequately describe signs of toxicity or efficacy. However, various studies have demonstrated that these techniques are both safe and effective in large cohorts of children. The PRAN database reported no cases of major complications like local anesthetic toxicity or permanent neurologic injury. The most common issues that came up included pericatheter leakage, dislodgement, and failed blockade.[7] With these minimal risks and the benefit of improved analgesia for over 3 days, the practice is growing in a number of pediatric centers, especially in those that provide care to sports medicine patients.

Interestingly, the onset of the COVID-19 pandemic has increased the utilization of home peripheral nerve catheters. One institution saw a 3-fold increase with the start of COVID compared with their single-shot nerve block cohort.[38] Our hospital experienced a surge in patients with COVID occupying hospital beds. With this bed shortage, many elective surgeries that would normally require an inpatient admission were canceled, or postponed. However, many injuries that were elective became time-sensitive which made for a challenging situation for patients. Providers began using continuous nerve blocks to discharge patients home from the recovery room and, therefore, bypass the admission process. The outcomes were so positive that even with the resolution of the bed shortages, providers have continued their utilization of this practice.[39]

With greater use of ambulatory catheters, it will be vital to compare various analgesic approaches in the perioperative period. Not only is there a need for comparative efficacy studies but also for trials, examining long-term functional outcomes such as muscle strength, rehabilitation, and return to sports in patients getting regional anesthesia.

CLINICS CARE POINTS

- When planning for regional anesthetics in children, it is safe to perform them under general anesthesia.
- Although there is a lot of controversy around regional anesthetics masking the signs of compartment syndrome, the data have not supported this notion.

- Adolescents are a unique population that has a risk of prescription drug misuse, so continuous regional anesthetic techniques should strongly be considered to reduce opioid consumption after surgery.

DISCLOSURE

Dr W. Alrayashi has no disclosures to report; Dr R. Brusseau has no disclosures to report. Dr J. Cravero has no disclosures to report.

REFERENCES

1. Jain NB, Higgins LD, Losina E, et al. Epidemiology of musculoskeletal upper extremity ambulatory surgery in the United States. BMC Musculoskelet Disord 2014; 15(1):4.
2. Oladeji AK, Minaie A, Landau AJ, et al. Blood loss in hip reconstructive surgery in children with cerebral palsy: when do I need to be prepared for blood transfusion? J Pediatr Orthop B 2022. https://doi.org/10.1097/bpb.0000000000000926.
3. Rudra A, Chatterjee S, Sengupta S, et al. The child with cerebral palsy and anaesthesia. Indian J Anaesth 2008;52(4):397–403.
4. Ponde V. Recent trends in paediatric regional anaesthesia. Indian J Anaesth 2019;63(9):746–53.
5. Tsui B, Suresh S. Ultrasound imaging for regional anesthesia in infants, children, and adolescents: a review of current literature and its application in the practice of extremity and trunk blocks. Anesthesiology 2010;112(2):473–92.
6. Walker BJ, Long JB, Sathyamoorthy M, et al. Complications in Pediatric Regional Anesthesia: an Analysis of More than 100,000 Blocks from the Pediatric Regional Anesthesia Network. Anesthesiology 2018;129(4):721–32.
7. Ecoffey C, Lacroix F, Giaufre E, et al, Association des Anesthesistes Reanimateurs Pediatriques d'Expression F. Epidemiology and morbidity of regional anesthesia in children: a follow-up one-year prospective survey of the French-Language Society of Paediatric Anaesthesiologists (ADARPEF). Paediatr Anaesth 2010;20(12):1061–9.
8. Longacre MM, Cummings BM, Bader AM. Building a bridge between pediatric anesthesiologists and pediatric intensive care. Anesth Analg 2019;128(2): 328–34.
9. Lonnqvist PA. Asleep or awake: is paediatric regional anaesthesia without general anaesthesia possible? Br J Anaesth 2020;125(2):115–7.
10. Giaufre E, Dalens B, Gombert A. Epidemiology and morbidity of regional anesthesia in children: a one-year prospective survey of the French-Language Society of Pediatric Anesthesiologists. Anesth Analg 1996;83(5):904–12.
11. Ivani G, Suresh S, Ecoffey C, et al. The european society of regional anaesthesia and pain therapy and the american society of regional anesthesia and pain medicine joint committee practice advisory on controversial topics in pediatric regional anesthesia. Reg Anesth Pain Med 2015;40(5):526–32.
12. Lin JA, Blanco R, Shibata Y, et al. Advances of techniques in deep regional blocks. Biomed Res Int 2017;2017:7268308.
13. Davis ET, Harris A, Keene D, et al. The use of regional anaesthesia in patients at risk of acute compartment syndrome. Injury 2006;37(2):128–33.
14. Klucka J, Stourac P, Stouracova A, et al. Compartment syndrome and regional anaesthesia: critical review. Biomed Pap Med Fac Univ Palacky Olomouc Czech Repub 2017;161(3):242–51.

15. Tuckey J. Bilateral compartment syndrome complicating prolonged lithotomy position. Br J Anaesth 1996;77(4):546–9.
16. Nathanson MH, Harrop-Griffiths W, Aldington DJ, et al. Regional analgesia for lower leg trauma and the risk of acute compartment syndrome: Guideline from the Association of Anaesthetists. Anaesthesia 2021;76(11):1518–25.
17. Lonnqvist PA, Ecoffey C, Bosenberg A, et al. The European society of regional anesthesia and pain therapy and the American society of regional anesthesia and pain medicine joint committee practice advisory on controversial topics in pediatric regional anesthesia I and II: what do they tell us? Curr Opin Anaesthesiol 2017;30(5):613–20.
18. Uzel AP, Steinmann G. Thigh compartment syndrome after intramedullary femoral nailing: possible femoral nerve block influence on diagnosis timing. Orthop Traumatol Surg Res 2009;95(4):309–13.
19. Marhofer P, Halm J, Feigl GC, et al. Regional anesthesia and compartment syndrome. Anesth Analgesia 2021;133(5):1348–52.
20. Steen KH, Issberner U, Reeh PW. Pain due to experimental acidosis in human skin: evidence for non-adapting nociceptor excitation. Neurosci Lett 1995;199(1):29–32.
21. Raja S, Meyer R, Ringkamp M, et al. Peripheral neural mechanisms of nociception. In: Wall PMR, editor. Textbook of pain. Philadelphia, PA: Churchill Livingston; 1999. p. 31–4.
22. Soo B, Howard JJ, Boyd RN, et al. Hip displacement in cerebral palsy. J Bone Joint Surg Am 2006;88(1):121–9.
23. Robin J, Graham HK, Baker R, et al. A classification system for hip disease in cerebral palsy. Dev Med Child Neurol 2009;51(3):183–92.
24. Shrader MW, Jones J, Falk MN, et al. Hip reconstruction is more painful than spine fusion in children with cerebral palsy. J Child Orthop 2015;9(3):221–5.
25. Zhou L, Willoughby K, Strobel N, et al. Classifying Adverse Events Following Lower Limb Orthopaedic Surgery in Children With Cerebral Palsy: reliability of the Modified Clavien-Dindo System. J Pediatr Orthop 2018;38(10):e604–9.
26. Medical Advisory S. Intrathecal baclofen pump for spasticity: an evidence-based analysis. Ont Health Technol Assess Ser 2005;5(7):1–93.
27. Von Korff M, Saunders K, Thomas Ray G, et al. De facto long-term opioid therapy for noncancer pain. Clin J Pain 2008;24(6):521–7.
28. Boretsky K, Hernandez MA, Eastburn E, et al. Ultrasound-guided lumbar plexus block in children and adolescents using a transverse lumbar paravertebral sonogram: Initial experience. Paediatr Anaesth 2018;28(3):291–5. https://doi.org/10.1111/pan.13328.
29. Eklund SE, Staffa SJ, Alrayashi W, et al. COVID-19 pandemic as impetus for sustained utilization of home peripheral nerve catheter program. Paediatr Anaesth 2022;32(3):482–4. https://doi.org/10.1111/pan.14383.
30. Piper NA, Flack SH, Loeser JD, et al. Epidural analgesia in a patient with an intrathecal catheter and subcutaneous pump to deliver baclofen. Paediatr Anaesth 2006;16(9):989–92.
31. Eklund SE, Samineni AV, Koka A, et al. Epidural catheter placement in children with baclofen pumps. Pediatr Anesth 2021;31(2):178–85.
32. Liu DV, Lin YC. Current Evidence for Acute Pain Management of Musculoskeletal Injuries and Postoperative Pain in Pediatric and Adolescent Athletes. Clin J Sport Med 2019;29(5):430–8.
33. Garofoli M. Adolescent substance abuse. Prim Care 2020;47(2):383–94.

34. Hassan MM, Rahman OF, Hussain ZB, et al. Opioid overprescription in adolescents and young adults undergoing hip arthroscopy. J Hip Preserv Surg 2021; 8(1):75–82.
35. Visoiu M, Joy LN, Grudziak JS, et al. The effectiveness of ambulatory continuous peripheral nerve blocks for postoperative pain management in children and adolescents. Paediatr Anaesth 2014;24(11):1141–8.
36. Ilfeld BM, Morey TE, Enneking FK. The delivery rate accuracy of portable infusion pumps used for continuous regional analgesia. Anesth Analg 2002;95(5):1331–6.
37. Tawfic QA, Freytag A, Armstrong K. A survey of acute pain service in Canadian teaching hospitals. Braz J Anesthesiology 2021;71(2):116–22.
38. Susan EE, Walid A, Roland S, et al. COVID-19 Pandemic as Impetus for Sustained Utilization of Home Peripheral Nerve Catheter Program. Paediatr Anaesth 2021;32(3):482–4.
39. Jones MR, Petro JA, Novitch MB, et al. Regional catheters for outpatient surgery-a comprehensive review. Curr Pain Headache Rep 2019;23(4):24.

Acute Extremity Compartment Syndrome and (Regional)

Anesthesia: The Monster Under the Bed

José A. Aguirre, MD, MSc[a,c,]*, Morné Wolmarans, MD[b],
Alain Borgeat, MD[c,d]

KEYWORDS

- Acute compartment syndrome • Regional anesthesia • Extremity • Complication
- Tissue pressure

KEY POINTS

- Acute compartment syndrome (ACS) is a devastating posttrauma/surgery complication, which can lead to permanent disability of upper and lower extremities
- The clinical signs/symptoms for ACS are unreliable. The use of intracompartmental pressure measurement is necessary to confirm the diagnosis of ACS.
- Continuous peripheral regional anesthesia is an effective technique for postoperative analgesia of upper and lower extremities.
- The main factors for adverse outcome after ACS are delays in definitive diagnosis (compartment pressure measurement) and surgical management (fasciotomy).
- A review of the literature emphasizes breakthrough pain, present in most described cases, as the most important clinical sign.
- Continuous neuraxial anesthesia might produce dense motor and sensory blocks and has the potential to delay the diagnosis of ACS. Caution is warranted.
- The application of local anesthetics at low concentrations through peripheral regional catheter, intra-articular analgesia, (continuous) fascial plane blocks, and sensory blocks is considered effective and safe means to provide analgesia for trauma/postsurgical patients at risk for ACS.

[a] Institute of Anaesthesiology, Triemli City Hospital Zurich, Birmensdorferstrasse 497, 8063 Zürich, Switzerland; [b] Department of Anesthesia, Norfolk and Norwich University Hospital NHS Trust, Regional Anesthesia UK (RA-UK), Colney Lane, Norwich NR4 7UY, UK; [c] Balgrist Campus, Lengghalde 5, 8008 Zürich, Switzerland; [d] Department of Surgery, University of Illinois at Chicago, 402 CSB MC 958840 South Wood Street, Chicago, IL 60612, USA
* Corresponding author.
E-mail address: josealejandro.aguirre@stadtspital.ch

Anesthesiology Clin 40 (2022) 491–509
https://doi.org/10.1016/j.anclin.2022.06.001
1932-2275/22/© 2022 Elsevier Inc. All rights reserved.

Abbreviations	
CEDA	continuous epidural anesthesia
EDA	epidural anesthesia
ESP	erector spinae block
PCEA	patient controlled epidural analgesia
PECS	pectoral nerve block
QLB	quadratus lumborum block
TCI	target controlled anesthesia
TAP	transversus abdominis block

THE HISTORY OF COMPARTMENT SYNDROME

Volkmann[1] described in 1881 myonecrosis and secondary contracture after prolonged muscle ischemia. He suspected that limb splints caused muscle cell death due to diminished arterial blood flow, describing an untreated compartment syndrome. Bardenheuer[2] reported in 1911 the first forearm compartment decompression for impending compartment syndrome, and Griffiths[3] published in 1940 patients developing Volkmann's contractures after embolectomy of the brachial artery. He was the first to introduce the 5 P's of compartment syndrome (pain, pallor, paresthesias, paralysis, pulselessness) in clinical practice. Whitesides and colleagues[4] described the effects of time on muscle survival in compartment pressure, demonstrating that less than 5% of muscle cells were damaged after 4 hours of ischemia, whereas nearly 100% were damaged after 8 hours of ischemia. In a cadaveric forearm model, Havig and colleagues[5] demonstrated that fasciotomy is the decisive intervention to return the compartment pressures to normal values.

DEFINITION OF ACUTE COMPARTMENT SYNDROME

ACS is defined as an increase of pressure within a fixed osteofascial anatomic space, leading to an impairment of cellular function due to decreased local tissue perfusion and, when sustained, to irreversible damage to the contents of the compartment (nerves, muscles).[6] There are 3 variables (factors) affecting the outcome in the case of elevated compartment pressure: (1) how high is the pressure, (2) how long is the elevated pressure sustained, and (3) how severe are concomitant injuries? Classification systems should consider the most important variables in this progressive tissue injury: time and pressure, as described by Leversedge and colleagues.[7] It is important to note that the physiologic pressures vary between 8 mm Hg in adults and 10 to 15 mm Hg in children.[8,9]

Traditionally, an absolute pressure value of 30 mm of Hg was taken as a cutoff value, above which intervention was required. However, the difference in the diastolic pressure and intracompartmental pressure is used more reliably because compartment pressure depends on perfusion or the systemic blood pressure. According to Whitesides and Heckman[10] compartment syndrome occurs when the pressure increases up to 20 mm Hg below the diastolic pressure. Some investigators recommend an intervention when the delta pressure (ΔP = diastolic pressure − intracompartmental pressure) is less than 30 mm Hg considering this value (30 mm Hg) as diagnostic.[11]

CAUSE AND RISK FACTORS

Data from the Royal Infirmary of Edinburgh show an average annual incidence of 3.1 per 100,000 people (7.3 per 100,000 men and 0.7 per 100,000 women).[12] ACS is more

---

Box 1
Causes of compartment syndrome

External compression
- Constriction by casts, splint, pneumatic antishock garments
- Excessive traction to fractures
- Early surgical closure of fascial defects
- Third-degree burns (thermal, electric)

Secondary increased compartment pressure
- Iatrogenic injection
- Infiltrated intravenous catheters/inadvertent intra-arterial drug injection
- Intracompartmental hemorrhage
  - Bleeding after injury
  - Spontaneous bleeding due to hereditary bleeding disorders
  - Anticoagulant therapy
- Trauma from fractures (open or closed), osteotomies, vessel laceration
- Intramedullary nailing
- Gunshot
- Soft tissue trauma
- Prolonged positioning during surgery (lithotomy position)
- Crush injuries
- Ergotamine ingestion
- Drug overdose
- Prolonged tetany
- Intraosseous fluid administration in children
- Use of pumps during arthroscopy
- Postischemic
  - Ischemia reperfusion (after embolectomy, clamping of arteries, and so on)
  - Tourniquet
- Arterial injury/arterial spasm
- Tissue edema after snakebite
- Thrombosis/embolization
- Limb reimplantation

Modified from Tollens et al.[97]

---

common in males and in patients younger than 35 years.[13] Forty percent of all cases of ACS derive from tibial shaft fracture, 23% from soft tissue tibial trauma, and 18% from forearm fractures.[14] The Scottish series report that 36% of all tibial fractures and 23.2% of all blunt soft tissue injuries are associated with ACS.[12]

Children have a higher preexisting compartment pressure, but the ACS incidence in children is lower.[15] In the case of soft tissue damage, ACS can also occur in the absence of fractures. Factors associated with an increased risk of ACS after trauma are medical comorbidities associated with abnormal bleeding diatheses (clotting disorders, the use of anticoagulants), volume resuscitation, altered mental status, or neurologic compromise diminishing sensitivity and sensibility of the limbs[12] (**Box 1**).

PATHOPHYSIOLOGY OF COMPARTMENT SYNDROME

The pathophysiology of the compartment syndrome is complex. In this syndrome fluid shifts from the blood to the extracellular and intracellular space leading to an increased tissue pressure within the compartment. This shift leads to a decrease of capillary blood flow and a decrease in tissue Po_2 and ends in a metabolic deficit resulting in muscle ischemia and necrosis. When tissue pressures reach the threshold of 30 to 40 mm Hg[16] the extraluminal pressure causes progressive arteriole collapse and

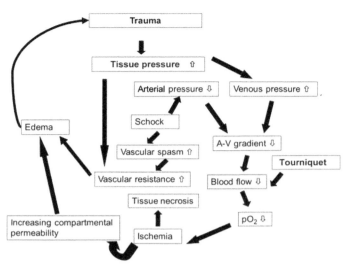

Fig. 1. Pathophysiology and the vicious circle of the acute compartment syndrome. (*Modified from* Janzing HM.[98])

local tissue hypoxia occurs with secondary shunting to areas with less vascular resistance. Dahn and colleagues[17] showed that local tissue perfusion stopped when the interstitial tissue pressure equals the diastolic blood pressure. Cell hypoxia is thus related to diminished arteriolar flow, venous obstruction, and a decreased arteriovenous gradient (**Fig. 1**).

There are 2 generally well-accepted pathophysiology theories:

- The arteriovenous gradient theory[18] and
- The ischemia-reperfusion syndrome[18,19]

Both theories advocate the increasing tissue pressure, the resulting decreasing capillary blood flow, and the decrease of tissue Po_2 with the end result of a metabolic deficit.

However, the latter hypothesis focuses on free radicals, calcium, and vasoactive substrates released under ischemic conditions resulting in the increased vessel permeability and subsequent increase in extravascular fluid and pressure. Both theories agree that the excess compartment pressure can only be rectified by creating the ability for the tissues to expand by fasciotomy.

DIAGNOSIS

The most important tool for diagnosis of an ACS is to keep a high index of clinical suspicion, especially in high-risk cases. However, signs and symptoms can be ambiguous leading to a late diagnosis of ACS.[18] Diagnosis becomes even more difficult in obtunded patients after a polytrauma, in the presence of equivocal clinical findings, after head injury with unconsciousness, and under perioperative narcotics or regional anesthesia (RA), where the clinical picture can be obscured.

Clinical Diagnosis of Acute Compartment Syndrome

The main clinical symptom of a developing ACS is considered to be pain. Palpable tension, paresthesia, paresis, and pulselessness might also be associated with ACS (**Box 2**). However, none of the commonly used signs in clinical practice is neither

---

Box 2
Symptoms and signs of acute compartment pressure

Symptoms:
- Pain is greater than expected or increasing
- Increase in pain and analgesic demand
- No relief after splinting or removal of casts
- Paresthesia in affected extremity

Signs:
- Pain on palpation/passive stretching of the affected compartment
- Tense and swollen compartment
- Sensory deficit of the nerves enclosed in the compartment
- Muscle weakness
- Pallor
- Pulselessness

CAVE:
   Usually pulses are present in the early stage of compartment and absent in late stage.
   Caution: Acute compartment syndrome can occur with palpable pulses.
   - Normal capillary refill present during early development of acute compartment syndrome.
   - Open fractures do not protect from acute compartment syndrome.
   - Clinical signs are of unclear value due to their low specificity and sensitivity
   Suggested clinical signs (in the case of RA or opioid PCA):
   - Breakthrough pain despite well-working RA
   - Increase demand of analgesics

Abbreviation: PCA, patient-controlled analgesia.

Modified from Torrero et al.[21]

---

reliable nor sufficiently specific or sensitive.[20] Pulselessness has to be considered a late sign with bad prognosis indicating muscle death with consequent need for radical surgery and severe disability.[14,20–23] Pain is also unreliable.[14,22] Moreover, Badhe and colleagues[24] described 4 cases of ACS of the lower extremity after trauma and surgery without considerable pain reported from the patients. Even the clinical palpation of the tense and swollen extremity as diagnostic criteria for detecting ACS has been shown to be strongly assessor dependent and unreliable with sensitivity of 24% and specificity of 55%[25] (**Table 1**).

Technical Diagnosis of Acute Compartment Syndrome

The most useful diagnostic method to decide if fasciotomy is indicated is the measurement of interstitial tissue pressures.

Although previous studies have reported that resting interstitial tissue pressures in the healthy vary between 0 and 8 mm Hg for the dorsal and volar forearm

---

Table 1
Accuracy of clinical signs for the diagnosis of acute compartment syndrome[20]

Sensitivity	13%–19%
Specificity	97%–98%
Positive predictive value	11%–15%
Negative predictive value	97%–98%
Probability of ACS if 1 clinical syndrome present	25%
Probability of ACS if 3 clinical syndromes present	93%

compartments and less than 15 mm Hg in the interosseous muscles of the hand,[26,27] several investigators have reported the diagnostic accuracy of different methods of pressure measurement if properly used. Interstitial tissue pressure measurements of noninjured forearms showed statistically significant differences over distances of only 4 cm.[26] Measurements performed at varying distances from a fracture showed statistically significant differences in pressure, with higher pressures within 5 cm of the fracture.[28] These findings illustrate the importance of proper placement of the needle for pressure monitoring.

In a case series of 116 consecutive patients, of whom 3 required fasciotomy, the use of a ΔP of less than or equal to 30 mm Hg as a threshold for fasciotomy led to no missed cases of ACS, no unnecessary fasciotomies, and no complications in any patients.[29]

The disadvantage to these measurements is that using both absolute and ΔP thresholds can result in high false-positive rates of up to 82%.[30]

Several studies have analyzed the reliability of various techniques for measuring compartment pressures. Boody and Wongworawat[31] compared different measurement equipment and concluded that side-port needles and slit catheters were more accurate than straight needles and that the arterial line manometer was the most accurate device. The Stryker device was also very accurate, but the Whitesides manometer apparatus was not precise enough for clinical use.[31]

An interesting development in noninvasive measurement techniques was introduced by the near-infrared spectroscopy (NIRS), which detects changes and trends in relative oxygen saturation of hemoglobin.[32,33] Using the Beer-Lambert law this technique profits from different light absorption properties to calculate concentrations of oxygenated and deoxygenated hemoglobin.

Adding spatial configuration, this method can measure changes in local muscle oxygen saturation and thus has the potential to detect and provide continuous monitoring of intracompartmental ischemia and hypoxia.[34] For noninvasive continuous monitoring NIRS has been labeled as safe and useful.[35] However, more studies are warranted to define how well NIRS correlates with critical pressure thresholds, considering limits to its penetration depth.

TREATMENT AND OUTCOME

When the suspicion of an incipient compartment syndrome is raised, often following clinical assessment, sometimes followed by invasive compartment pressure measurement, re-evaluation must be frequently performed and accurately documented.[7] Casts and circumferential dressings must be removed and positioning with tension or distortion must be avoided to not further compromise blood flow. Fluid therapy must be carefully evaluated, and electrolytes, renal function, and coagulation parameters carefully monitored.

Once the diagnosis of ACS has been established, the only available treatment is a surgical decompression of the affected osteofascial compartments.[36] Adequate decompression must be ascertained by direct visualization of the muscle groups while passively moving. After fasciotomy and judicious excision of nonviable tissue has been performed, a careful search for separate subcompartments should be undertaken.[37]

The essential factors for the outcome after fasciotomy seem to be the timing and the concomitant injuries.

Delaying fasciotomy for more than 12 hours has been shown to significantly worsen outcome.[28,38,39] According to Hayakawa and colleagues[40] fasciotomy performed within 6 hours after diagnosis of ACS led to a satisfactory outcome in 88% of the cases with an amputation rate of 3.2% and mortality rate of 2%, whereas fasciotomy after 12 hours showed satisfactory outcome in only 15% of cases, with 14% amputations and 4.3% deaths. There is sparse data about the time frame of greater than 6 hours but less than 12 hours, because residual deficits also occur if fasciotomy time is only 2 hours after ACS diagnosis.[41]

Considering medicolegal aspects, Bhattacharyya and Vrahas[42] reported 19 claims between 1980 and 2003. Ten claims were resolved in favor of the physician. Increasing time from the onset of symptoms to the fasciotomy was linearly associated with an increased indemnity payment ($P < .05$). A fasciotomy performed within 8 hours after the first presentation of symptoms was uniformly associated with a successful defense.[42]

ANESTHESIA AND COMPARTMENT SYNDROME
The Role of Regional Anesthesia

RA in patients with trauma or in patients at risk for development for ACS is a highly controversial topic, and a point of eternal contention between anesthesiologists and orthopedic and trauma surgeons.[43–45] However, there is no randomized trial comparing the clinical outcome of patients at risk of ACS who receive RA or do not. The actual clinical practice is based on narrative and often biased reviews of case reports, retrospective case series, recommendations, and reviews and differs from institution to institution.[22] Widely held beliefs suggest that the relief of postoperative pain and the sensory blockade from RA can mask ACS,[14,22,42–44] and therefore RA should be completely avoided.

However, the recently published guidelines from the Association of Anaesthetists of Great Britain and Ireland (AAGBI) on lower leg trauma and the risk of ACS[46] clearly state that good analgesia is a basic human right. Further recommendations from this guideline include early identification of patients at risk of developing ACS, multidisciplinary management protocols, and appropriate equipment for intercompartment pressure monitoring, with appropriately trained staff and protocols to deal with abnormal measurements. Single-shot spinal anesthesia, with the addition of an opioid, and single-shot or continuous peripheral nerve blocks (PNBs) using lower concentrations of local anesthetic drugs without adjuvants are not associated with delays in diagnosis, as long as appropriate postinjury and postoperative surveillance is used, including objective scoring charts.

In addition, both the European and the American Societies of Regional Anesthesia clearly acknowledge the lack of evidence-based data supporting the notion that RA increases the risk of delayed ACS diagnosis in children.[47] Data from the American College of Surgeons National Surgical Quality Improvement Project also show no differences in postoperative complications after lower extremity traumatic fractures between patients who received regional and general anesthesia.[48] Finally, large case series in which regional blocks were used for analgesia during extremity trauma surgery did not report cases of compartment syndrome.[49]

Few reviews concentrate on different techniques or types of RA and ACS,[22,50,51] and some present a collection of published literature for peripheral and central blocks.[15,52,53]

This review compiles all the information for the upper and lower extremities including central blocks, discussing the role of different techniques of RA and their impact on the diagnosis of ACS according to existing literature and offering acceptable practical solutions for safe RA practice.

Intravenous Regional Anesthesia and Compartment Syndrome

Different reports have implicated intravenous RA (IVRA) in causing ACS.[54–58] The most debated theories on the pathogenesis center on the double tourniquet required for this technique and cite ischemia-reperfusion injury with hyperemia, swelling, and the administration of high volumes of local anesthetics and adjuvants into a "newly created compartment."[55] The latter theory could not be confirmed in a volunteer study that showed no compartment pressure increase after IVRA with 1.5 mL/kg saline.[58] However, this study was not performed on fractured extremities, which limits its relevance to trauma care. Moreover, inflation pressure and duration have also been implicated as tourniquet-related factors of compartment syndrome.

Neuraxial Blocks and Lower Limb Compartment Syndrome

Anesthesia

There are no published case reports implicating single-shot epidural or single-shot spinal anesthesia in ACS. Although many investigators state that epidural analgesia does not contribute to delay the diagnosis of ACS,[59–67] epidural anesthesia and analgesia has still been implicated in masking symptoms of ACS leading to a delay in diagnosis.[22]

In most of the published cases epidural anesthesia was considered to have masked clinical symptoms of ACS such as pain.[22,50,68] Mar and colleagues[22] reviewed 23 cases in which epidural anesthesia (EDA) was supposed to have masked ACS and showed that in 90% the classical symptoms of ACS were actually present but not recognized soon enough. Breakthrough pain, which is a clear clinical indicator for an ACS, was present in most cases. In 4 cases the diagnosis of ACS was masked by a dense block caused by EDA, blunting the occurrence of breakthrough pain.

Peripheral Nerve Blocks and Compartment Syndrome

Anesthesia

No randomized study analyzing the effects of single shot or even continuous peripheral RA on ACS has been published. Only case reports or case series of varying quality[22,69–71] that have been subject of case scenarios[72] and of recent reviews are available.

Moreover, to date there is no case report confirming a diagnosis delay of ACS after RA of the upper extremity[72–75]; this is of importance because contrary to the lower limb, the upper extremity can be completely blocked with a single nerve block. For the lower extremities, 2 or 3 peripheral blocks are required for a complete limb block; this could reduce the probability that PNB masks an ACS, for example, if a saphenous nerve block is applied to provide analgesia to the tibia plateau, while the muscular compartments below the knee are not affected, owing to their innervation by the sciatic nerve. However, some of the published case reports have wrongly implicated a PNB for an ACS in a territory that was blocked, demonstrating that PNB could not be the cause for delaying ACS diagnosis.[69]

In other cases, breakthrough pain as a sign of an incipient ACS was simply ignored for hours delaying the diagnosis and early therapy for ACS.[76,77]

Since the widespread use of adjuvants prolonging analgesia, single-shot perineural blocks are becoming more popular for anesthesia or as combination to general anesthesia.[78] Ganeshan and colleagues[75] reported the case of a 75-year-old patient with a complicated forearm fracture receiving an axillary brachial plexus block (without a description of the type, volume, and concentration of the local anesthetic solution) for ambulatory internal fixation of the radius. Subsequently, the patient was discharged pain free and comfortable, but developed a compartment syndrome during the next 24 hours with a loss of sensation in the fingers, multiple swelling over the forearm and hand, and loss of motor function of the fingers. He was readmitted after

24 hours and a fasciotomy was performed.[75] In this case the signs of ACS were obviously present after the block had worn off.

Local anesthetics and postoperative analgesia

The duration of motor and sensory block clearly depends on the local anesthetic, the concentration, and the volume used. Motor block duration up to 20 hours for bupivacaine 0.5% has been described.[79] Sensory blocks usually last from 12.5 hours for ropivacaine 0.5% to 16 hours for levobupivacaine 0.33%.[80] The introduction of ultrasound for peripheral RA has shown that the volumes for block performance can be reduced leading to a shortening of the block time: 9.9 hours for ropivacaine 0.75%[81] and 106 to 185 minutes for lidocaine 1.5% with or without epinephrine.[82]

Furthermore, shortening of motor and sensory block can be achieved by using intermediate-acting agents like mepivacaine (up to 5 hours block duration) or even short-acting agents like lidocaine with or without additives (up to 5.5 hours block duration with epinephrine).[83] Chloroprocaine 3% has been shown to produce a sensory blockade of 101 to 112 minutes depending on the block performed and is a valid alternative.[84]

Continuous perineural blocks offer many advantages compared with single-shot RA concerning better postoperative pain therapy and avoidance of rebound pain.[85] Moreover, ACS can be confounded with rebound pain after a single-shot RA. Clinical evaluation of the patient is essential for a correct diagnosis.

Source of possible concern might be a prolonged loss of motor or sensory function for hours with the risk of masking clinical symptoms of ACS. Even after stopping or reducing an infusion of CPB, a sensory block may take 2 to 4 hours to recover. If the time frame of 6 hours for intervention shall be the standard then this delay has to be avoided. The idea of performing CPB with higher volumes and lower concentrations has led to a higher incidence of insensate limbs in some studies, but these findings have not been reproduced by all investigators. On the other hand, reducing the volume and augmenting the concentration has been shown to influence the incidence of pain.[86] Unfortunately, reduction of the ropivacaine concentration to 0.1%, as used for the walking epidural analgesia in obstetrics, has been shown to be inadequate for knee arthroplasty and hand surgery.[87] The catheter infusion should be started with a low concentration bolus of 10 to 20 mL ropivacaine 0.1% to 0.2% to avoid initial motor function loss, and continued with a continuous infusion (or patient controlled infusion) using ropivacaine 0.2% (4–6 mL/h, bolus 3–4 mL, lock out 20–30 min). Ropivacaine 0.3% does not influence motor strength more than 0.2% for interscalene block while offering improved opioid-sparing effects and could be used for continuous infusion after extremely painful surgery after an initial anesthetic bolus.[88]

Intra-articular and Single-Shot/Continuous Wound Infusion for Extremity Surgery

Continuous wound (articular) infusion (CWI) or periarticular infiltration (local infiltration analgesia [LIA]) has no impact on motor or major sensory block because it does not affect major nerves but improves postoperative analgesia.[89,90] The best evidence for LIA is in total knee arthroplasty, whereas other indications such as hip surgery and upper extremity trauma are less clear.[91]

There is no case report blaming LIA or CWI of delaying diagnosis of ACS.

Compartment/Fascial Plane Blocks

Fascial plane blocks are a new way of providing RA, where high volumes of usually low concentrated local anesthetics are applied to offer analgesia avoiding central blocks or PNBs. Fascial plane block leads to minimal, if at all, motor block and offers an interesting alternative for patients at risk for ACS. Subsartorial block of the saphenous nerve for medial tibia plateau fractures, supraumbilical fascia iliaca block for femur neck fractures, and quadratus lumborum blocks for hip fractures could become alternatives to classic PNBs in these patients.[92]

There is no case report blaming fascial plane blocks of delaying diagnosis of ACS.

DISCUSSION

To the best of our knowledge, case reports blaming single-shot or continuous PNB for the upper limb, single-shot or continuous PNB for the lower limb, single-shot EDA or spinal anesthesia, or continuous spinal anesthesia were rather missed diagnosis than masking symptoms of ACS. The remaining reports concentrate on continuous EDA for the lower limb.[15,22,52,53]

If well documented, almost all published cases showed that patient complained about increasing pain despite RA,[70] loss of motor function despite reduction of local anesthetic concentration,[68] or increasing analgesic demand.[22] Only in 4 cases in literature, a dense motor block after EDA at the time of diagnosis was observed.[93,94] Nerve blocks have been blamed for masking ACS in a territory the block did not even theoretically cover.[69] Some case reports did not give any details about documentation and/or patient management before start of symptoms/clinical signs.[22] Therefore, RA can only be considered to be associated, but not the cause in diagnosis delay.

Despite these considerations, the use of RA for patients at risk for ACS remains a topic of dispute between anesthetists and surgeons.[44] As reported by Cascio and colleagues[95] a good, standardized documentation improves the awareness of this complex diagnosis. The investigators found in a retrospective study of preoperative medical records of 30 consecutive patients who underwent fasciotomies for ACS that documentation was inadequate in 21 (70%) patient records.[41]

Proper documentation and a high level of suspicion coupled with postoperative repeated clinical and, if needed, invasive monitoring are of utmost importance.[37,41] Data must be recorded at least at 2-hour interval; in the case of new or pathologic findings, the frequency of assessment must be adapted. The classical 5 P's (see **Box 2**, **Table 1**) is of unreliable value[20] particularly in the presence of RA, and should therefore be complemented by the clinical signs breakthrough pain and increasing analgesic demand.[50] As described by Bae and colleagues[96] an increase in analgesic need preceded neurovascular changes by an average of 7.3 hours (range 0–30). A compartment syndrome must be excluded at this point.[96]

SUGGESTED CLINICAL PRACTICE FOR THE USE OF REGIONAL ANESTHESIA IN PATIENTS AT RISK FOR ACUTE COMPARTMENT SYNDROME

Based on the literature presented in this review and following the recommendations of the latest guideline from the AAGBI,[46] the use of RA is a safe option if surgeons, anesthesiologists, and nurses in the post anesthesia care unit (PACU) and wards keep a high index of suspicion and have the knowledge how to document, diagnose, and treat ACS. Multidisciplinary protocols, objective scoring charts, patient consent, and senior surgical colleague consensus should be documented to provide every patient with a satisfactory analgesia plan.

As previously done per case scenario, the authors present an updated version of possible concepts for anesthesia and analgesia management of patients at risk for ACS[72] (**Table 2**).

Table 2

Recommendation for anesthesia and postoperative analgesia for patients at high risk for postoperative acute compartment syndrome

Anesthesia Techniques	Recommendation	Drugs to Be Used	Duration of Action	Comments
GA	Yes if not high-risk patient. For analgesia combine preferably with Lc-CPNB	Propofol/gas Low-dose long-acting opioids (fentanyl); remifentanil until Lc-CPNB	Remifentanil: 5 min after TCI is stopped	Consider central blocks additional to GA only postoperative pain is an issue that cannot be controlled with peripheral nerve blocks or systemic drugs. If used, use short- medium-acting local anesthetics to allow motoric recovery after surgery
SSPA	Consider pharmacology of LA relevant to duration to surgery time	Bupivacaine 0.5% hyperbaric/ isobaric low dose (7.5–max 10 mg) If needed add: fentanyl/morphine/clonidine Chloroprocaine 1% 50 mg Prilocaine 2% hyperbaric/isobaric 30–60 mg	Bupivacaine: 3–4 h Mepivacaine: 2–3 h Chloroprocaine: 1–2 h Prilocaine: 1.5–2.5 h	No case report related to ACS. Consider unilateral SSPA for shorter duration. Avoid combination with continuous EDA
CSPA	No if GA possible No if SSPA possible Yes if GA contraindicated and surgery longer as duration of SSPA (+additives)	Surgery: Bupivacaine isobaric or hyperbaric 0.5% during surgery 0.5–2 mL initial bolus, thereafter adaptation to surgery time and sensory level Analgesia: Bupivacaine isobaric 0.125%–0.2% for 0.5–1 mL/h	Bupivacaine: 2–3.5 h, depending on the intraoperative titration	No case report related to ACS. Start the analgesia with the lowest concentration and increase the sensory level just to cover the site of surgery. Close documented monitoring (every hour) during infusion

(continued on next page)

Table 2
(continued)

Anesthesia Techniques	Recommendation	Drugs to Be Used	Duration of Action	Comments
Single-shot epidural (EDA)	No if GA possible. Consider combination with SSPA (CSE). Yes if GA contraindicated and drugs can be adapted to surgical time	Ropivacaine 0.75%–1% Lidocaine 1.5% Chloroprocaine 3%	Ropivacaine: 3–6h Lidocaine: 3.5 h Chloroprocaine: 2.5 h	No case report related to ACS. Avoid combination with continuous EDA
Continuous epidural (CEDA)	No if GA possible No if postoperative analgesia is possible with CPNB Yes in rare *exceptions Lc-CEDA*	Ropivacaine 0.1% (–0.2%) Levobupivacaine 0.125% If needed add sufentanil 1 μ/mL, fentanyl 1–3 μ/mL)	During infusion and 2–4 h after infusion stop Wash out with 30 mL saline leads to block resolution within 60 min	Avoid EDA whenever possible. Many case reports, although only 4 with dense motor block associated with ACS. Close documented monitoring (every hour) during infusion. Consider wash out. No PCEA
SPNB	Only if postoperative pain is minimal and only if local anesthetics can be adapted to surgery time *Lc-CPNB is the better choice*	Lidocaine 1.5% Mepivacaine 1% Chloroprocaine 2%–3% Ropivacaine 0.2%	Lidocaine: 2.5–3 h Mepivacaine: 2–4 h Chloroprocaine: 1–2 h	Case reports for the lower extremity (but ACS signs ignored)
CPNB	Yes if catheter placement possible without previous block or short-duration PNB	Ropivacaine: bolus with 10–20 mL of 0.1%–0.2% PCRA: ropivacaine 0.1%–0.2% (0.3%) 4-6 mL/h, bolus 3-4 mL, lock out 20–30 min	During infusion and 30–60 min after infusion stop. Motor function typically not impaired with these dosages	Case reports for the lower extremity (but ACS signs ignored). If possible avoid initial bolus, or perform it with the lowest concentration. PCRA or CPNB possible. 0.3% only if pain problem after exclusion of ACS

Continuous wound/ intra-articular infusion (LIA)	Yes	Ropivacaine 0.2%–0.3% Bupivacaine 0.25%	Covers pain only during infusion; for single-shot analgesia up to 24 h	For lower extremity not inferior to PNB, for upper extremity unclear data, PNB probably more effective
Fascia plane blocks (FIB, ESP, TAP, QLB, PECS)	Yes	Ropivacaine 0.2%–0.3% Bupivacaine 0.25%	Depending on location, volume, and concentration	No association with missed ACS. As no (reduced) resulting motor block, good alternative for pain treatment

Abbreviations: CPNB, continuous perineural block; CSPA, continuous spinal anesthesia; CSE, combined spinal and epidural anesthesia; GA, general anesthesia; LA, local anesthetics; Lc, low concentration; LIA, local infiltration analgesia; max, maximum; PCRA, patient-controlled regional anesthesia; SPNB, single-shot PNB; SSPA, single-shot spinal anesthesia.[72]

- Anesthesia
  - General anesthesia should be avoided if there are clear advantages for RA but limitation of block duration relative to surgery time should be considered to avoid a dense and long-lasting sensory and motor block.
  - IVRA should be avoided in cases at risk for ACS.
  - Spinal anesthesia for surgery is a good option to avoid general anesthesia. Long-acting drugs (bupivacaine 0.5%) should be used only for surgeries greater than 90 minutes; otherwise advantage of prilocaine 2% or chloroprocaine 1% should be taken for shorter surgeries. The addition of spinal opioids may also be considered. Continuous spinal anesthesia or combinations with EDA (combined spinal and epidural anesthesia) are indicated only for cases in which general anesthesia is contraindicated.
- Analgesia
  - Intraoperative LIA or CWI are good analgesia regimens for upper and lower extremities and have no implication regarding motor function.
  - Fascial plane blocks using dilute local anesthetics offer good analgesia, and their effect can be extended using catheters. Similarly, here, there is almost no impact on motor function.
  - Continuous central nerve blocks are only indicated when no PNB can be performed; they can produce a dense sensory and motor block and are the only blocks that have been shown to mask the diagnosis of ACS. If used, lowest possible concentrations (ropivacaine 0.1%–0.2%) should be applied.
  - PNBs are the preferred method for analgesia but need thorough postoperative documentation and follow-up by the pain team. Again, the lowest possible concentrations with higher flow rates should be used to avoid dense motor blocks. Even top-ups over the catheter should be performed with low concentration (ropivacaine 0.2%–0.3%) and higher volumes (20 mL). Caution: A top-up need can be a sign of ACS!

CLINICS CARE POINTS

In the clinical findings, paralysis and pulselessness are already late sings of an ACS

- The only safe way to exclude or proof an ACS is the measurement of the compartment pressure.
- Breakthrough pain described as a pain that suddenly overcharges the ongoing pain therapy (peripheral regional anesthesia or intravenous opioids) is a serious sign for an ACS.

DISCLOSURE

The authors have nothing to disclose.

REFERENCES

1. Volkmann R. Die ischaemischen Muskellaehmungen und Kontrakturen. Centralbl Chir 1881;(8):801–3.
2. Bardenheuer L. Die Entstehung und Behandlung der ischaemischen Muskelkontraktur und Gangraen. Deutsche Zeitschrift F Chir 1911;108:44.
3. Griffiths DL. Volkmann's ischaemic contracture. Br J Surg 1940;(28):239–60.

4. Whitesides TE, Haney TC, Morimoto K, et al. Tissue pressure measurements as a determinant for the need of fasciotomy. Clin Orthop Relat Res 1975;113:43–51.
5. Havig MT, Leversedge FJ, Seiler JG 3rd. Forearm compartment pressures: an in vitro analysis of open and endoscopic assisted fasciotomy. J Hand Surg 1999;24(6):1289–97.
6. Friedrich JB, Shin AY. Management of forearm compartment syndrome. Hand Clin 2007;23(2):245–54.
7. Leversedge FJ, Moore TJ, Peterson BC, et al. Compartment syndrome of the upper extremity. J Hand Surg 2011;36(3):544–59.
8. Shadgan B, Menon M, O'Brien PJ, et al. Diagnostic techniques in acute compartment syndrome of the leg. J Orthop Trauma 2008;22(8):581–7.
9. Staudt JM, Smeulders MJ, van der Horst CM. Normal compartment pressures of the lower leg in children. J Bone Joint Surg Br 2008;90(2):215–9.
10. Whitesides TE, Heckman MM. Acute compartment syndrome: update on diagnosis and treatment. J Am Acad Orthop Surg 1996;4(4):209–18.
11. Duckworth AD, Mitchell SE, Molyneux SG, et al. Acute compartment syndrome of the forearm. J Bone Joint Surg Am 2012;94(10):e63.
12. McQueen MM, Gaston P, Court-Brown CM. Acute compartment syndrome. Who is at risk? J Bone Joint Surg Br 2000;82(2):200–3.
13. Martin JT. Compartment syndromes: concepts and perspectives for the anesthesiologist. Anesth Analg 1992;75(2):275–83.
14. Elliott KG, Johnstone AJ. Diagnosing acute compartment syndrome. J Bone Joint Surg Br 2003;85(5):625–32.
15. Klucka J, Stourac P, Stouracova A, et al. Compartment syndrome and regional anaesthesia: critical review. Biomed Pap Med Fac Univ Palacky Olomouc Czech Repub 2017;161(3):242–51.
16. Ashton H. Critical closure in human limbs. Br Med Bull 1963;19:149–54.
17. Dahn I, Lassen NA, Westling H. Blood flow in human muscles during external pressure or venous stasis. Clin Sci 1967;32(3):467–73.
18. Bodansky D, Doorgakant A, Alsousou J, et al. Acute Compartment Syndrome: Do guidelines for diagnosis and management make a difference? Injury 2018;49(9): 1699–702.
19. Bulkley GB. Pathophysiology of free radical-mediated reperfusion injury. J Vasc Surg 1987;5(3):512–7.
20. Ulmer T. The clinical diagnosis of compartment syndrome of the lower leg: are clinical findings predictive of the disorder? J Orthop Trauma 2002;16(8):572–7.
21. Torrero JI, Aroles F. Effect of intramedullary nails in tibial shaft fractures as a factor in raised intracompartmental pressures: a clinical study. Eur J Trauma Emerg Surg 2009;35:553–61.
22. Mar GJ, Barrington MJ, McGuirk BR. Acute compartment syndrome of the lower limb and the effect of postoperative analgesia on diagnosis. Br J Anaesth 2009; 102(1):3–11.
23. Kosir R, Moore FA, Selby JH, et al. Acute lower extremity compartment syndrome (ALECS) screening protocol in critically ill trauma patients. J Trauma 2007;63(2): 268–75.
24. Badhe S, Baiju D, Elliot R, et al. The 'silent' compartment syndrome. Injury 2009; 40(2):220–2.
25. Shuler FD, Dietz MJ. Physicians' ability to manually detect isolated elevations in leg intracompartmental pressure. J Bone Joint Surg Am 2010;92(2):361–7.
26. Seiler JG 3rd, Womack S, De L'Aune WR, et al. Intracompartmental pressure measurements in the normal forearm. J Orthop Trauma 1993;7(5):414–6.

27. Ardolino A, Zeineh N, O'Connor D. Experimental study of forearm compartmental pressures. J Hand Surg 2010;35(10):1620–5.
28. Heckman MM, Whitesides TE Jr, Grewe SR, et al. Compartment pressure in association with closed tibial fractures. The relationship between tissue pressure, compartment, and the distance from the site of the fracture. J Bone Joint Surg Am 1994;76(9):1285–92.
29. McQueen MM, Court-Brown CM. Compartment monitoring in tibial fractures. The pressure threshold for decompression. J Bone Joint Surg Br 1996;78(1):99–104.
30. Nelson JA. Compartment pressure measurements have poor specificity for compartment syndrome in the traumatized limb. J Emerg Med 2013;44(5): 1039–44.
31. Boody AR, Wongworawat MD. Accuracy in the measurement of compartment pressures: a comparison of three commonly used devices. J Bone Joint Surg Am 2005;87(11):2415–22.
32. Arbabi S, Brundage SI, Gentilello LM. Near-infrared spectroscopy: a potential method for continuous, transcutaneous monitoring for compartmental syndrome in critically injured patients. J Trauma 1999;47(5):829–33.
33. Shuler MS, Reisman WM, Kinsey TL, et al. Correlation between muscle oxygenation and compartment pressures in acute compartment syndrome of the leg. J Bone Joint Surg Am 2010;92(4):863–70.
34. Rolfe P. In vivo near-infrared spectroscopy. Annu Rev Biomed Eng 2000;2: 715–54.
35. Widder S, Ranson MK, Zygun D, et al. Use of near-infrared spectroscopy as a physiologic monitor for intra-abdominal hypertension. J Trauma 2008;64(5): 1165–8.
36. Shadgan B, Menon M, Sanders D, et al. Current thinking about acute compartment syndrome of the lower extremity. Can J Surg 2010;53(5):329–34.
37. Kashuk JL, Moore EE, Pinski S, et al. Lower extremity compartment syndrome in the acute care surgery paradigm: safety lessons learned. Patient Saf Surg 2009; 3(1):11.
38. Geary N. Late surgical decompression for compartment syndrome of the forearm. J Bone Joint Surg Br 1984;66(5):745–8.
39. Janzing H, Broos P, Rommens P. Compartment syndrome as a complication of skin traction in children with femoral fractures. J Trauma 1996;41(1):156–8.
40. Hayakawa H, Aldington DJ, Moore RA. Acute traumatic compartment syndrome: a systematic review of results of fasciotomy. Trauma 2009;11:5–35.
41. Cascio BM, Pateder DB, Wilckens JH, et al. Compartment syndrome: time from diagnosis to fasciotomy. J Surg Orthop Adv 2005;14(3):117–21 [discussion: 120-111].
42. Bhattacharyya T, Vrahas MS. The medical-legal aspects of compartment syndrome. J Bone Joint Surg Am 2004;86-A(4):864–8.
43. Davis, ET, Harris A, Keene D, et al. The use of regional anaesthesia in patients at risk of acute compartment syndrome. Injury 2006;37(2):128–33.
44. Thonse R, Ashford RU, Williams TI, et al. Differences in attitudes to analgesia in post-operative limb surgery put patients at risk of compartment syndrome. Injury 2004;35(3):290–5.
45. Gregoretti C, Decaroli D, Miletto A, et al. Regional anesthesia in trauma patients. Anesthesiol Clin 2007;25(1):99–116, ix-x.
46. Nathanson MH, Harrop-Griffiths W, Aldington DJ, et al. Regional analgesia for lower leg trauma and the risk of acute compartment syndrome: guideline from the Association of Anaesthetists. Anaesthesia 2021;76(11):1518–25.

47. Ivani G, Suresh S, Ecoffey C, et al. The European Society of Regional Anaesthesia and Pain Therapy and the American Society of Regional Anesthesia and Pain Medicine Joint Committee Practice Advisory on Controversial Topics in Pediatric Regional Anesthesia. Reg Anesth Pain Med 2015;40(5):526–32.
48. Brovman EY, Wallace FC, Weaver MJ, et al. Anesthesia type is not associated with postoperative complications in the care of patients with lower extremity traumatic fractures. Anesth Analg 2019;129(4):1034–42.
49. Zadrazil M, Opfermann P, Marhofer P, et al. Brachial plexus block with ultrasound guidance for upper-limb trauma surgery in children: a retrospective cohort study of 565 cases. Br J Anaesth 2020;125(1):104–9.
50. Johnson DJ, Chalkiadis GA. Does epidural analgesia delay the diagnosis of lower limb compartment syndrome in children? Paediatr Anaesth 2009;19(2):83–91.
51. Mannion S, Capdevila X. Acute compartment syndrome and the role of regional anesthesia. Int Anesthesiol Clin 2010;48(4):85–105.
52. Marhofer P, Halm J, Feigl GC, et al. Regional Anesthesia and Compartment Syndrome. Anesth Analg 2021;133(5):1348–52.
53. Driscoll EB, Maleki AH, Jahromi L, et al. Regional anesthesia or patient-controlled analgesia and compartment syndrome in orthopedic surgical procedures: a systematic review. Local Reg Anesth 2016;9:65–81.
54. Guay J. Adverse events associated with intravenous regional anesthesia (Bier block): a systematic review of complications. J Clin Anesth 2009;21(8):585–94.
55. Ananthanarayan C, Castro C, McKee N, et al. Compartment syndrome following intravenous regional anesthesia. Can J Anaesth 2000;47(11):1094–8.
56. Maletis GB, Watson RC, Scott S. Compartment syndrome. A complication of intravenous regional anesthesia in the reduction of lower leg shaft fractures. Orthopedics 1989;12(6):841–6.
57. Hastings H 2nd, Misamore G. Compartment syndrome resulting from intravenous regional anesthesia. J Hand Surg Am 1987;12(4):559–62.
58. Mabee JR, Bostwick TL, Burke MK. Iatrogenic compartment syndrome from hypertonic saline injection in Bier block. J Emerg Med 1994;12(4):473–6.
59. Beerle BJ, Rose RJ. Lower extremity compartment syndrome from prolonged lithotomy position not masked by epidural bupivacaine and fentanyl. Reg Anesth 1993;18(3):189–90.
60. Dunwoody JM, Reichert CC, Brown KL. Compartment syndrome associated with bupivacaine and fentanyl epidural analgesia in pediatric orthopaedics. J Pediatr Orthop 1997;17(3):285–8.
61. Goldsmith AL, McCallum MI. Compartment syndrome as a complication of the prolonged use of the Lloyd-Davies position. Anaesthesia 1996;51(11):1048–52.
62. Heyn J, Ladurner R, Ozimek A, et al. Gluteal compartment syndrome after prostatectomy caused by incorrect positioning. Eur J Med Res 2006;11(4):170–3.
63. Iwasaka H, Itoh K, Miyakawa H, et al. Compartment syndrome after prolonged lithotomy position in patient receiving combined epidural and general anesthesia. J Anesth 1993;7(4):468–70.
64. Llewellyn N, Moriarty A. The national pediatric epidural audit. Paediatr Anaesth 2007;17(6):520–33.
65. Montgomery CJ, Ready LB. Epidural opioid analgesia does not obscure diagnosis of compartment syndrome resulting from prolonged lithotomy position. Anesthesiology 1991;75(3):541–3.
66. Stotts AK, Carroll KL, Schafer PG, et al. Medial compartment syndrome of the foot: an unusual complication of spine surgery. Spine (Phila Pa 1976) 2003;28(6):E118–20.

67. Tuckey J. Bilateral compartment syndrome complicating prolonged lithotomy position. Br J Anaesth 1996;77(4):546–9.
68. Hailer NP, Adalberth G, Nilsson OS. Compartment syndrome of the calf following total knee arthroplasty–a case report of a highly unusual complication. Acta Orthop 2007;78(2):293–5.
69. Hyder N, Kessler S, Jennings AG, et al. Compartment syndrome in tibial shaft fracture missed because of a local nerve block. J Bone Joint Surg Br 1996; 78(3):499–500.
70. Uzel AP, Steinmann G. Thigh compartment syndrome after intramedullary femoral nailing: possible femoral nerve block influence on diagnosis timing. Orthop Traumatol Surg Res 2009;95(4):309–13.
71. Uzel AP, Lebreton G, Socrier ML. Delay in diagnosis of acute on chronic exertional compartment syndrome of the leg. Chir Organi Mov 2009;93(3):179–82.
72. Aguirre JA, Gresch D, Popovici A, et al. Case scenario: compartment syndrome of the forearm in patient with an infraclavicular catheter: breakthrough pain as indicator. Anesthesiology 2013;118(5):1198–205.
73. Sermeus L, Boeckx S, Camerlynck H, et al. Postsurgical compartment syndrome of the forearm diagnosed in a child receiving a continuous infra-clavicular peripheral nerve block. Acta Anaesthesiol Belg 2015;66(1):29–32.
74. Rauf J, Iohom G, O'Donnell B. Acute compartment syndrome and regional anaesthesia - a case report. Rom J Anaesth Intensive Care 2015;22(1):51–4.
75. Ganeshan RM, Mamoowala N, Ward M, et al. Acute compartment syndrome risk in fracture fixation with regional blocks. BMJ Case Rep 2015. https://doi.org/10.1136/bcr-2015-210499. pii. bcr2015210499.
76. Munk-Andersen H, Laustrup TK. Compartment syndrome diagnosed in due time by breakthrough pain despite continuous peripheral nerve block. Acta Anaesthesiol Scand 2013;57(10):1328–30.
77. Cometa MA, Esch AT, Boezaart AP. Did continuous femoral and sciatic nerve block obscure the diagnosis or delay the treatment of acute lower leg compartment syndrome? A case report. Pain Med 2011;12(5):823–8.
78. Albrecht E, Kern C, Kirkham KR. A systematic review and meta-analysis of perineural dexamethasone for peripheral nerve blocks. Anaesthesia 2015;70(1): 71–83.
79. Fanelli G, Casati A, Beccaria P, et al. A double-blind comparison of ropivacaine, bupivacaine, and mepivacaine during sciatic and femoral nerve blockade. Anesth Analg 1998;87(3):597–600.
80. Gonzalez-Suarez S, Pacheco M, Roige J, et al. Comparative study of ropivacaine 0.5% and levobupivacaine 0.33% in axillary brachial plexus block. Reg Anesth Pain Med 2009;34(5):414–9.
81. Gautier P, Vandepitte C, Ramquet C, et al. The minimum effective anesthetic volume of 0.75% ropivacaine in ultrasound-guided interscalene brachial plexus block. Anesth Analg 2011;113(4):951–5.
82. Harper GK, Stafford MA, Hill DA. Minimum volume of local anaesthetic required to surround each of the constituent nerves of the axillary brachial plexus, using ultrasound guidance: a pilot study. Br J Anaesth 2010;104(5):633–6.
83. Kuntz F, Bouaziz H, Bur ML, et al. [Comparison between 1.5% lidocaine with adrenaline and 1.5% plain mepivacaine in axillary brachial plexus block]. Ann Fr Anesth Reanim 2001;20(8):693–8.
84. Khy V, Girard M. [The use of 2-chloroprocaine for a combined lumbar plexus and sciatic nerve block]. Can J Anaesth 1994;41(10):919–24.

85. Abdallah FW, Halpern SH, Aoyama K, et al. Will the Real Benefits of Single-Shot Interscalene Block Please Stand Up? A Systematic Review and Meta-Analysis. Anesth Analg 2015;120(5):1114–29.

86. Ilfeld BM, Moeller LK, Mariano ER, et al. Continuous peripheral nerve blocks: is local anesthetic dose the only factor, or do concentration and volume influence infusion effects as well? Anesthesiology 2010;112(2):347–54.

87. Paauwe JJ, Thomassen BJ, Weterings J, et al. Femoral nerve block using ropivacaine 0.025%, 0.05% and 0.1%: effects on the rehabilitation programme following total knee arthroplasty: a pilot study. Anaesthesia 2008;63(9):948–53.

88. Borgeat A, Aguirre J, Marquardt M, et al. Continuous interscalene analgesia with ropivacaine 0.2% versus ropivacaine 0.3% after open rotator cuff repair: the effects on postoperative analgesia and motor function. Anesth Analg 2010; 111(6):1543–7.

89. Liu SS, Richman JM, Thirlby RC, et al. Efficacy of continuous wound catheters delivering local anesthetic for postoperative analgesia: a quantitative and qualitative systematic review of randomized controlled trials. J Am Coll Surg 2006; 203(6):914–32.

90. Aguirre J, Baulig B, Dora C, et al. Continuous epicapsular ropivacaine 0.3% infusion after minimally invasive hip arthroplasty: a prospective, randomized, double-blinded, placebo-controlled study comparing continuous wound infusion with morphine patient-controlled analgesia. Anesth Analg 2011;114(2):456–61.

91. Yung EM, Got TC, Patel N, et al. Intra-articular infiltration analgesia for arthroscopic shoulder surgery: a systematic review and meta-analysis. Anaesthesia 2021;76(4):549–58.

92. Chin KJ, Lirk P, Hollmann MW, et al. Mechanisms of action of fascial plane blocks: a narrative review. Reg Anesth Pain Med 2021;46(7):618–28.

93. Somayaji HS, Hassan AN, Reddy K, et al. Bilateral gluteal compartment syndrome after total hip arthroplasty under epidural anesthesia. J Arthroplasty 2005;20(8):1081–3.

94. Tang WM, Chiu KY. Silent compartment syndrome complicating total knee arthroplasty: continuous epidural anesthesia masked the pain. J Arthroplasty 2000; 15(2):241–3.

95. Cascio BM, Pateder DB, Farber AJ, et al. Improvement in documentation of compartment syndrome with a chart insert. Orthopedics 2008;31(4):364.

96. Bae DS, Kadiyala RK, Waters PM. Acute compartment syndrome in children: contemporary diagnosis, treatment, and outcome. J Pediatr Orthop 2001;21(5): 680–8.

97. Tollens T, Janzing H, Broos P. The pathophysiology of the acute compartment syndrome. Acta Chir Belg 1998;98(4):171–5.

98. Janzing HM. Epidemiology, Etiology, Pathophysiology and Diagnosis of the Acute Compartment Syndrome of the Extremity. Eur J Trauma Emerg Surg 2007;33(6): 576–83.

Blood Conservation Techniques and Strategies in Orthopedic Anesthesia Practice

Richa Sharma, MBBS, Yolanda Huang, MD, Anis Dizdarevic, MD*

KEYWORDS

- Orthopedic surgery • Blood conservation • Patient blood management
- Orthopedic anesthesia • Anemia management • Tranexamic acid

KEY POINTS

- Select orthopedic surgery procedures carry an increased risk of bleeding and need for blood transfusion.
- Patient blood management strategies involve preoperative anemia management, transfusion guidelines, restrictive hemoglobin triggers, surgical and anesthesia technique advances, and use of antifibrinolytics to reduce bleeding and transfusion rates.
- Perioperative anticoagulant optimization and management is patient- and surgery-specific and based on risk–benefit balance between thromboembolic events and bleeding.
- Careful intraoperative blood pressure management is an important component of anesthesia care that plays role in reduction of surgical bleeding.
- Tranexamic acid is effective in decreasing blood loss and need for transfusion with favorable patient safety profile.

INTRODUCTION

Orthopedic surgery procedures, which have been increasing in numbers globally and are among the most common surgical procedures performed, have traditionally been associated with relatively significant intraoperative and postoperative bleeding and need for blood transfusion.[1–4] The risk of bleeding and resulting blood transfusion is especially high and relevant in total hip arthroplasty (THA) and total knee arthroplasty (TKA), spinal deformity correction and instrumentation procedures, trauma and oncological procedures involving long bones and pelvis, and more complex revision

The authors have nothing to disclose.
Department of Anesthesiology, Columbia University Irving Medical Center, 622 West 168th Street, PH 5, New York, NY 10032, USA
* Corresponding author.
E-mail address: ad2689@cumc.columbia.edu
Twitter: @Drsharma_richa (R.S.)

Anesthesiology Clin 40 (2022) 511–527
https://doi.org/10.1016/j.anclin.2022.06.002
1932-2275/22/© 2022 Elsevier Inc. All rights reserved.
anesthesiology.theclinics.com

procedures. Establishing and maintaining adequate surgical hemostasis is extremely important, but due to the combination of patient- and surgery-specific factors, meeting this goal successfully may often be challenging. Notwithstanding years of significant advances in safety protocols, blood transfusions could still be associated with complications, including allergic reactions, transfusion-related acute lung injury, transfusion-related circulatory volume overload, infection, thromboembolic events, as well as prolonged hospitalization, increased morbidity and mortality, and increased costs.[5,6]

Efforts have been made to develop and study methods to decrease surgical bleeding and reduce unnecessary blood transfusion, and according to the recent reports, there has been significant decline in red blood cell (RBC) and plasma transfusions nationally among hospitalized patients in the United States through 2018.[7]

Patient blood management (PBM) programs, involving preoperative anemia management, transfusion guidelines, restrictive hemoglobin (Hb) triggers, clinical decision and education initiatives, as well as advances in surgical techniques, anesthesia practice, blood conservation, and use of antifibrinolytic therapy, have been associated with reduced blood use, less complications, and similar or improved clinical outcomes.[8,9]

This review describes the comprehensive up-to-date perioperative approaches used in orthopedic anesthesiology practice to optimize patient care, minimize blood loss, and reduce blood transfusion rates.

PREOPERATIVE STRATEGIES

PBM is a patient-centered, multidisciplinary approach aimed to provide a perioperative management plan to improve patient outcomes.[10,11] For surgical patients, the three pillars of PBM are: active diagnosis and management of preoperative anemia, utilization of surgical, anesthesia, and pharmacologic methods to minimize operative blood loss, and, lastly, optimization of patient's physiological tolerance of postoperative anemia. A meta-analysis conducted by Althoff and colleagues[12] showed a comprehensive PBM program is associated with reduced transfusion need of red blood cells as well as lower complication and mortality. A retrospective study involving orthopedic surgery showed that the implementation of PBM in patients undergoing total joint arthroplasty was associated with lower allogeneic blood transfusion (ABT), decreased length of stay and all-cause, 90-day, readmission.[13]

Anemia Management

Optimizing erythropoiesis, stated in the first pillar of PBM, can be done preoperatively by detecting and treating anemia. Anemia is defined by the World Health Organization (WHO) as Hb less than 12 g/dL in adult nonpregnant women and less than 13 g/dL in adult men. In the surgical setting, preoperative anemia was detected in a third of patients undergoing major elective surgery in Spain, and, of the approximate 1300 patients undergoing orthopedic surgery, 26% were anemic.[14] Multiple studies in the United States showed preoperative anemia prevalence range from 19% to 45.6% in general orthopedic surgery patients, including those with hip fractures.[15,16] Preoperative anemia when left untreated can lead to adverse intraoperative and postoperative outcomes, such as acute kidney injury, stroke, myocardial infarction, and death.[17] Preoperative anemia is an independent predictor for 30-day mortality in noncardiac surgery[18] as well as long-term mortality in orthopedic surgeries.[19] Therefore, it is prudent to assess and optimize patient's red blood cell mass when elective surgery is planned. Vaglio and colleagues recommended that elective major orthopedic surgery should be postponed until the underlying etiology of anemia had been investigated and treated.[20]

A panel of physicians convened by the Network for Advancement of Transfusion Alternatives recommended patients undergoing elective orthopedic surgery to have an Hb level determined 28 days before the scheduled procedure if possible.[21] If there is any presence of anemia defined by the WHO criteria, further evaluation is warranted to diagnose and treat the underlying etiology before elective surgery.[21,22] The causes of anemia include iron, folate, and B12 deficiencies, chronic renal insufficiency, anemia of chronic inflammation (formerly known as anemia of chronic disease), and unexplained anemia. Once anemia is detected on screening, further laboratory testing to assess iron status, storage and synthetic capacity can assist in the algorithmic approach to most patient management, excluding those with hereditary hemoglobinopathies.[21,23] To distinguish between different forms of anemia, levels of serum ferritin (SF) and transferrin saturation (TS) are evaluated.

Iron Deficiency

The concentration of extracellular ferritin found in serum is used as an indirect biomarker to estimate body iron storage. However, ferritin is an acute phase reactant and can be elevated in an inflammation state. The TSAT level reflects circulating iron available for erythropoiesis and is calculated by the serum iron concentration divided by the total iron-binding capacity of transferrin. In the absence of inflammation, SF less than 30 μg/L is the most sensitive and specific test used to identify absolute iron deficiency. When concomitant inflammatory state is present (C-reactive protein > 5 mg/L), SF less than 100 μg/L or TSAT less than 20% is indicative of iron deficiency.

If iron storage is sufficient (SF > 100 μg/L), the next step is to determine whether the patient has concurrent chronic kidney disease based on laboratory values of serum creatinine and glomerular filtration rate. Often patients with chronic kidney disease have functional iron deficiency. It is characterized by laboratory findings of SF 100 to 500 μg/L and TSAT less than 20%, where there is inadequate mobilization of iron despite normal or elevated iron stores in the setting of increased demands. If the iron status and kidney function are both normal in patients, then the etiology of anemia can be attributed to either anemia of inflammation or vitamin B12 and/or folate deficiency. The direct measurement of serum vitamin B12 and folate can delineate the difference. Patients with anemia of inflammation have laboratory findings of low TSAT with normal-to-elevated SF and high hepcidin levels. Inflammation causes the upregulation of hepatic hepcidin levels which leads to internalization and degradation of iron exporter ferroportin, resulting in iron sequestration and low plasma iron levels.

Treatment of Anemia

Patient with absolute iron deficiency anemia should be treated with iron supplementation. If causes from low iron intake or decreased intestinal iron absorption are ruled out, patient should receive a workup for the source of iron loss. If there is no obvious source of blood loss, a referral to a gastroenterologist is warranted to eliminate gastrointestinal lesions as the source of insidious bleeding. 2018 PBM International Consensus Conference experts recommended that the decision on the route of iron administration should be based on the magnitude of anemia, time to surgical procedure and the ability to tolerate and absorb oral iron.[22] Oral iron of daily 40 to 60 mg or alternate-day 80 to 100 mg treatment should be initiated by primary care physician 6 to 8 weeks before surgery.[24] Drawbacks of oral iron are related to its common side effect of nausea, vomiting, constipation or diarrhea, and its poor bioavailability as the absorption can be inhibited by dietary iron chelators or by medications such as H2 blockers and proton-pump inhibitors.[25]

Patients with decreased intestinal iron absorption due to decreased absorptive surface (eg, celiac disease, postoperatively from gastrectomy, duodenal bypass, bariatric surgery) or altered pH (autoimmune atrophic gastritis, *Helicobacter pylori* infection) are candidates for intravenous iron supplementation. Other established indications for intravenous iron are patients with severe anemia (Hb < 7–8 g/dL), or those with functional iron deficiency and those with anemia of inflammation when not responding to erythropoiesis-stimulating agents. Dosage and frequency of intravenous iron infusion are dependent on the formulation. Iron gluconate and iron sucrose require repeated infusions, whereas iron isomaltoside, iron dextran, ferumoxytol, and ferric carboxymaltose can be administered in one or two infusions to replace the total iron deficit. Infusion reactions, ranging from mild/moderate (nausea, pruritis, urticaria, flushing) to severe (hypotension, dyspnea), should be monitored in patients. It is a relative contraindication for patients with infection to receive iron infusion, as iron can act as a growth factor for pathogen. Patients with nutritional deficiency from low folate or vitamin B12 can be supplemented with folic acid 1 mg/day or vitamin B12 1000 mcg/day via the oral route.[23]

Blood Transfusion Trigger

The trigger for red blood cell transfusion has traditionally been based on a convention of Hb level less than 10 g/L. The Transfusion Requirements in Critical Care study, a landmark, multicenter prospective randomized trial conducted in Canada, examined more than 800 intensive care patients randomized to either the standard, liberal transfusion trigger of Hb less than 10 g/L or the restrictive group of Hb less than 7 g/L. and showed no significant difference in the overall 30-day mortality between the two groups.[26] Subsequent studies and meta-analyses in various patient populations demonstrated that restrictive transfusion strategy had outcomes noninferior and perhaps even superior, as compared with a liberal transfusion strategy.[27–30] These transfusion trials lead to the incorporation of restrictive transfusion strategy in PBM, but it should also not shift our focus away from treating the underlying etiology of anemia. Implementation of restrictive transfusion strategy along with other PBM goals at a single center in orthopedic patients showed a reduction in the need for ABT and a decreased in the incidence of deep wound infection.[31] The 2018 PBM International Consensus Conference developed the conditional recommendations to adopt a restrictive transfusion threshold (Hb concentration less than 8 g/dL) in patients with cardiovascular disease and other risk factors undergoing surgery for hip fractures.[22] We should also exercise caution to not base our decision to transfuse on a single Hb value.

One fading practice of blood conservation strategies is preoperative autologous blood donation, which would eliminate the complications from allogenic blood transfusion and preserve the allogenic blood supply.[32] Patients' own blood donated before surgery, with frequency up to twice weekly and time frame up to 72 hours before surgery, can be stored for 6 weeks and used intraoperatively and postoperatively. However, given the logistical and cost constraints, potential unused waste, and the limited benefits shown in a meta-analysis,[33,34] routine practice of preoperative autologous blood donation is not advisable in elective orthopedic surgery.[35–37]

Perioperative Anticoagulant Optimization

Whether to initiate, continue, or stop antiplatelet or anticoagulant in surgical patients is a complex preoperative decision. Factors to consider when making such decision include (1) intraoperative bleeding risk of the surgical case, (2) perioperative thromboembolic risk of myocardial infarction, stroke, and deep vein thrombosis/pulmonary embolism, and (3) use of intraoperative anesthesia technique. Reducing perioperative bleeding risk by stopping anticoagulant medication fulfills the second goal of PBM but it needs to be balanced against the risk of thromboembolic events. Initial Perioperative Ischemic Evaluation 2 trial showed that administration of aspirin (ASA) during the surgical period has no effect on the composite outcome of death or nonfatal myocardial infarction at 30 days after noncardiac surgery (HR 0.99, 95% CI [0.86–1.15], P = 0.92); However, major bleeding was more common (HR 1.23, 95% CI [1.01–1.49], P = 0.04).[38] In patients taking ASA for primary prevention, it can be discontinued 7 to 10 days before surgery, but most consensus statements recommend continuing ASA for orthopedic surgery. For patients with stent implantation for coronary artery disease and who are on dual antiplatelet therapy of ASA and P2Y12 platelet receptor antagonist, it is recommended that elective noncardiac surgery be delayed at least 30 days after bare-metal stent implantation and ideally 6 months after drug-eluting stent (DES) implantation. Surgery may be considered after 3 months of DES implantation if the risk of delaying surgery outweighs the risk of stent thrombosis. ASA monotherapy should be continued if possible, and P2Y12 platelet receptor antagonist should be stopped 5 to 7 days before and restarted shortly after surgery.[39] The American Society of Regional Anesthesia and Pain Medicine (ASRA) suggests stopping clopidogrel 5-7 days before performing any neuraxial technique.[40] Direct oral anticoagulants (DOACs) have been developed to overcome the limitations of warfarin, which requires coagulation monitoring for dose adjustment. The discontinuation of DOACs should start at least 48 hours before surgery to decrease the risk of bleeding and 72 hours in patients with reduced creatinine clearance. If intraoperative neuraxial technique is desirable, ASRA guidelines recommend to discontinue rivaroxaban and apixaban 3 days and dabigatran 5 days before procedure.[40]

INTRAOPERATIVE STRATEGIES
Neuraxial Anesthesia in Total Hip and Knee Arthroplasty to Reduce Blood Loss

International Consensus on Anaesthesia-Related Outcomes after Surgery group established in 2019 that neuraxial anesthesia is the recommended primary anesthetic in hip and knee surgeries given comparable or lower postoperative negative outcomes when compared with general anesthesia (GA).[41] In 2006, two meta-analyses reported pooled data from randomized controlled trials (RCTs) showing statistically significant decrease in blood loss in patients undergoing THA and spinal fusions under neuraxial anesthesia versus GA.[42,43] A large retrospective study reported a 35.9% decrease in rates of intraoperative and postoperative blood transfusion in patients who received revision THA under neuraxial anesthesia relative to GA.[44] Yap and colleagues[45] demonstrated less blood loss and transfusion rates in patients who received neuraxial anesthesia for ambulatory, unilateral TKA or THA in a retrospective, multicenter study of 11,523 patients.

Regional Anesthesia

The benefits or lack thereof of peripheral nerve blocks on blood loss during orthopedic surgeries are not well established. In 2017, a non-blinded RCT of 40 patients who underwent TKA under spinal anesthesia and received either intrathecal morphine or a femoral infusion catheter plus single shot sciatic nerve block, showed significantly lower postoperative blood loss in the latter group.[46] They hypothesized a role of vasoconstrictive effects of ropivacaine in decreasing blood loss. Significant reduction in intraoperative and postoperative blood loss was demonstrated in a prospective, double-blinded RCT of 60 patients who underwent THA under GA with a posterior lumbar plexus block compared with those who did not receive the block.[47] The blood loss reduction was in addition to lower anesthetic requirements and mean arterial pressure observed. In a prospective study published in 2017 no difference in blood loss was found in GA versus cervical plexus block in anterior cervical discectomy and fusion surgery.[48] Malik and colleagues analyzed data from over 12,000 patients undergoing below knee amputations and reported a significantly decreased need for perioperative blood transfusions when regional anesthesia, over general, was used.[49] In an RCT involving patients undergoing THA under GA, sole local wound infiltration of ropivacaine-epinephrine did not produce decreased blood loss or transfusion requirements.[50]

Intraoperative Blood Pressure Regulation

Conduction of hypotensive anesthesia has long been used in orthopedic surgery for reduction of intraoperative blood loss. Pharmacologic and non-pharmacologic techniques and neuraxial anesthesia have been used to achieve deliberate hypotension (DH). Apart from limiting blood loss, reduction in operative time, decreased tissue edema from ligation or cautery and better myocardial performance have been shown with DH.[51,52] Paul and colleagues performed a meta-analysis of 17 RCTs involving seven THA, one TKA, one spinal fusion, and eight orthognathic surgeries in which methods of DH included sodium nitroprusside, volatile anesthetics, prostaglandin E1, epidural blockade, remifentanil, and propranolol. Despite significant heterogeneity, the study showed reduction in blood loss irrespective of the method used to achieve the hypotension.[53] The safety of DH has always been a concern especially in the geriatric population, or those with cardiovascular risk factors or comorbidities. Jiang and colleagues reported a reduction in intraoperative bleeding and blood transfusion volume and no increased rate of mortality in a meta-analysis of 30 studies pertaining to orthopedic surgeries in which DH was used.[54] However, most of the patients were healthy in their analysis, and they concluded that it was unclear whether or not DH was a safe technique to be routinely used for orthopedic surgery. The intraoperative approaches to DH include the utilization of antihypertensive medications, such as calcium channel and beta blockers, neuraxial, and GA. These approaches are specifically tailored to have relatively short duration with predictable, dose-dependent effect, and negligible consequences on vital organs. In patients undergoing TKA without the use of tourniquet and with tranexamic acid (TXA) administration, a prospective cohort study of 278 patients suggested a systolic blood pressure (SBP) of 90 to 100 mm Hg as optimal for reduction of blood loss and at the same time avoiding postoperative complications.[55] Although no specific large studies have established the safety of DH in the orthopedic population, multiple analyses have been undertaken to study the relation of hypotension and major adverse cardiac or cerebrovascular events (MACCE), kidney injury, and other composite serious outcomes. Wanner and colleagues randomized 458 patients undergoing major noncardiac surgeries to either have intraoperative mean arterial blood pressures (MAP) maintained to greater than 75 mm Hg or greater than 60 mm Hg, and reported no statistically significant difference in the incidence of immediately postoperative or longer term (up to 1 year) cardiovascular events or perioperative kidney injury between the two groups.[56] However, longer cumulative intraoperative hypotensive time with MAP less than 65 mm Hg could be associated with adverse events. Gregory and colleagues conducted a large multicenter retrospective cohort study of 368,222 noncardiac surgeries evaluating intraoperative blood pressure and MACCE. They reported a progressively increased association for MACCE and 30- and 90-day mortality for each absolute blood pressure threshold examined (MAP ≤ 75, ≤ 65, ≤ 55 mm Hg).[57] Similarly, a strong association between intraoperative hypotension and adverse postoperative outcomes were demonstrated by Wijnberge, Sessler and colleagues.[58–60] Consensus recommendations were put forth stating intraoperative MAP less than 60 to 70 mm Hg and SBP less than 100 mm Hg were associated with myocardial injury and death, and the former also with acute kidney injury (AKI) in adults having noncardiac surgery.[59] In addition to absolute MAP threshold lowering, it has also been recommended that MAP not be lowered more than 20 to 30% of the baseline during anesthesia (relative threshold). The duration of hypotension has also been suggested to be an important factor.

Temperature Regulation

Hypothermia has inhibitory effects on the coagulation cascade and platelet function and can be deleterious when uncontrolled, especially in the presence of acidosis and hypervolemia and has been studied in orthopedic surgery population.[61–64] Surgery and anesthesia, both GA and neuraxial, can result in perioperative hypothermia (PH) via multiple etiologies, including vasodilation, ambient room temperature effects, direct heat loss from patient body and surgical wound exposure, and impaired thermoregulation.[64] PH should be diligently minimized due to its many undesirable effects, such as predisposition to surgical site infections, increased risk of adverse postoperative cardiac events, impaired metabolism, postoperative shivering, and reduced patient satisfaction. Retrospective studies involving patients who underwent TKA and THA showed that intraoperative hypothermia was associated with intraoperative blood loss and perioperative transfusion rates.[61,62] Recent studies have established the association of hypothermia and bleeding and/or transfusion requirements in elderly patients with hip fractures and patients with pelvic and acetabular fractures.[65,66] However, other studies did not find adverse bleeding effects of relative intraoperative hypothermia in shoulder and spine surgeries, although operative time and surgery type were mentioned as possible confounders.[67,68] Intraoperative interventions to reduce the rate of PH use active body surface warming systems (ABSW), usually with intraoperative forced air warming or circulating water mattress, warming intravenous fluids, and prevention of heat loss with reflective blankets, limiting surface area exposed to the ambient environment, and heat and humidity exchanger in ventilator circuit. A Cochrane systematic review including 67 RCT looking at the effectiveness of ABSW, in most cases forced air warmers, in preventing PH, found blood loss and transfusion rates to be reduced due to clinically irrelevant amounts.[69]

Autologous Normovolemic Hemodilution

This technique involves withdrawal of blood immediately before or after the induction of anesthesia and replacement with either crystalloids or colloids to arrive at a target Hb value with the aim to decrease the amount of red blood cells lost as the surgery proceeds and to improve microcirculation.[70,71] The collected blood is transfused when the intraoperative blood loss has abated and if a certain lower threshold of hematocrit is reached. Two prospective comparative studies from India involving orthopedic and major head and neck surgeries examined the effect of either receiving or not receiving normovolemic hemodilution.[72,73] In both studies a significant decrease in transfusion requirements was noted in patients receiving autologous normovolemic hemodiluation, with less postoperative complications noted in one study. Li and colleagues performed a retrospective review of 120 patients who underwent lumbar spine fusion surgery.[74] They discovered that the intraoperative blood loss was significantly lower when TXA was given either with or without autologous normovolemic hemodilution (ANH), as compared with neither intervention. On the other hand, ANH alone did not produce statistically significant lower blood loss compared with control.

Cell Salvage Technique

Blood from the surgical field can be collected, processed such that the red blood cells are separated from the debris, and reintroduced into the patient's circulation. The benefits of this technique are to reduce allogenic blood transfusion and its associated complications, including alloimmunization, transmission of infectious diseases (especially in resource constrained parts of the world), and hemolytic and febrile transfusion reactions. The main downside is the costs associated with the cell salvage process and, if used postoperatively, the presence of multiple machines at the bedside make for a more cumbersome experience. In a 2010 Cochrane systematic review, cell salvage was found efficacious in reducing the need for allogeneic red cell transfusion in adult elective surgery, including orthopedic.[75] There was no increase in mortality, reoperation for bleeding, infection, wound complications, nonfatal myocardial infarction, thrombosis, and risk of stroke or length of hospital stay due to intraoperative or postoperative blood salvage, but rather a decrease in infection and wound complications. The benefit of intraoperative cell saver use in reducing the demand for allogenic blood transfusion was reported in scoliosis surgery, especially in patients starting with a low Hb, undergoing surgeries with long duration and/or significant blood loss.[76] A 2015 meta-analysis of over 43 studies found cell salvage to significantly reduce the RBC exposure rate and the volume of RBCs transfused in both THA and TKA.[77] However, conflicting data were presented by So-Osman and colleagues[78] in an RCT including 683 patients with a preoperative Hb level between 10 and 13 g/dL undergoing hip and/or knee arthroplasty where autologous blood salvage was not found to be effective in sparing erythrocyte transfusion, perhaps due to a relatively low blood loss overall and low volume of recovered blood.

Tranexamic Acid

TXA is one of the most extensively studied pharmaceutical agents with established benefits in multiple orthopedic surgeries.[79] Poeran and colleagues studied 872,416 patients from 510 hospitals in the United States and reported reduced odds for blood transfusion by more than 60%.[80] Patients who received TXA had lower rates of allogeneic or autologous transfusion, thromboembolic complications, overall complications, need for mechanical ventilation, and admission to an intensive care unit. Filingham and colleagues' also demonstrated that topical, IV, and oral TXA were all superior to placebo in decreasing blood loss and transfusion requirements in TJA with no clearly superior route among them.[81,82] Topical administration (joint irrigation or intra-articular instillation) of TXA is a viable option for patients with unknown or higher thrombotic risk.[83] Although direct increased risk has not been found in studies, concerns regarding prothrombotic adverse events including deep vein thrombosis, myocardial infarction, pulmonary embolism, and cerebrovascular events, especially in high-risk patients have been raised. Recent systematic reviews and meta-analysis did not find an association between TXA and venous thromboembolism (VTE), including venous thrombosis, cerebral, pulmonary and myocardial, ischemia and infarction irrespective of dosing and a known history of VTE.[84–86] TXA appeared more effective than other antifibrinolytics aprotinin and epsilon aminocaproic acid in spine surgeries, and any antifibrinolytic was better than placebo.[87] A recent meta-analysis of three somewhat heterogeneous studies demonstrated significantly decreased transfusion rates with TXA administration in patients who received acetabular or pelvic surgeries.[88] Pecold and colleagues conducted a meta-analysis of 10 studies, of which 7 were RCTs, looking at shoulder arthroplasties until December 2021.[89] They established the utility of TXA in reduction of perioperative blood loss among other benefits.

Desmopressin (DDAVP; 1-deamino-8-D-arginine-vasopressin) is a synthetic analog of vasopressin, which leads to a transient increase in plasma levels of factor VIII and Von Willebrand (VW) factor.

A 2017 Cochrane review examined the evidence for the efficacy of DDAVP in reducing blood loss in various orthopedic surgeries and showed transfusion rate was higher when patients received DDAVP as compared with TXA and an uncertain effect in the transfused blood volume when DDAVP was compared with placebo.[90]

Platelet-Rich Plasma

Plasma have been long known to be storehouses of multiple growth factors such as platelet-derived growth factor, insulin like growth factor, and transforming growth factor-beta. Supplementing the operative environment with thrombin-activated platelet-rich plasma (PRP) has been shown to enhance osteogenesis and promote hemostasis and functional recovery.[91–93] A meta-analysis of 12 studies did not show any benefit in reducing postoperative blood loss with the intraoperative use of PRP in TKA.[94] Ma and colleagues suggested that PRP might be effective in reducing postoperative blood loss and attenuating Hb drop without increasing the risks of postoperative complications after TKA, but the evidence was low.[95]

Thromboelastography

Thromboelastography (TEG) has been employed as a point-of-care test perioperatively to assess a patient's blood coagulation profile within minutes by testing the strength of an evolving clot over time. It has been used in situations where massive blood loss and potential for transfusions exists such as trauma, certain surgeries, and critical care to guide transfusion therapy. TEG gives clinicians the information about different components of the coagulation cascade and where the patient lies on the spectrum from hypo- to hypercoagulable. This makes transfusion of blood products more directed toward addressing the underlying abnormality and sometimes results in less overall products transfused.[96,97] Hagedorn and colleagues[98] shared a thorough review of TEG and its role in orthopedics. The utility of this test ranges from preoperatively predicting if the chances of spinal epidural hematoma with a neuraxial procedure may be high in the presence of innate or iatrogenic coagulopathies to postoperatively guiding anticoagulant use in a personalized fashion.[99–104] The central role of fibrinolysis as the reason for bleeding in scoliosis surgery was established by TEG.[105] Zhang and colleagues[106] also confirmed via TEG that administration of TXA in THA surgeries did not alter the coagulation profile of patients undergoing THA.

Tourniquet Use

Application of tourniquet during extremity surgeries significantly decreases blood flow to the operative area during the procedure and improves visualization of the surgical field. At the same time, it has also been linked to contribute to a hypercoagulable state and promote hemolysis perioperatively. Multiple recent meta-analyses and RCTs have suggested that although tourniquet use may decrease visible intraoperative blood loss, it may also contribute to an increase in the total blood loss as well as lead to other adverse effects.[107–109]

POSTOPERATIVE STRATEGIES

The risks of both perioperative bleeding as well as postoperative VTE in orthopedic patients, especially those undergoing hip and knee arthroplasty surgery, trauma and pelvic surgery, are relatively significant and dependent on both patient- and procedure-related risk factors.[110] The American College of Chest Physicians has estimated the combined baseline untreated risk of venous thromboembolism for 35 days after surgery to be 4.3%, with the highest risk occurring in the first 7 to 14 days. A systematic review of randomized trial by Chan and colleagues, comparing different pharmacologic thromboprophylaxis regimens in TKA and THA patients demonstrated that the symptomatic average VTE rate (1%) was similar to or exceeded by the average rate of major bleeding (0.5–2%) and combined clinically relevant bleeding (4–5%).[111] Risk stratification of orthopedic surgery patients, relying on patient- and surgery-specific factors, requires an important risk–benefit balance and applying the best options for safe and effective VTE prophylaxis. Recent approaches have been more individualized and studies have been focusing on symptomatic VTE as outcomes.[112]

Pharmacologic therapies used for VTE prophylaxis include ASA, low-molecular-weight heparin (LMWH), DOACs, or a combination of agents. They are surgery and patient tailored and initiated 6 to 12 hours after surgery if adequate hemostasis achieved. The American Society of Hematology guidelines recommend ASA and DOACs over LMWH for thromboprophylaxis after orthopedic surgery, whereas the National Institute for Health Care Excellence guidelines recommend LMWH or fondaparinux sodium as an alternative to ASA and DOACs.[113]

Antiplatelet therapies stopped preoperatively are usually resumed once adequate hemostasis is achieved and risk of further bleeding is minimal. Warfarin is restarted at the preoperative dosing schedule within the first 24 hours as well. Therapeutic bridging with LMWH and DOAC are restarted within 48 to 72 hours.[114,115]

SUMMARY

Strategies to minimize perioperative bleeding and blood transfusion in orthopedic surgery have been shown to improve patient outcomes and reduce health care cost. Interventions involve optimizing preoperative anemia, implementing restrictive blood transfusion thresholds, and using antifibrinolytic agents, in addition to advances in surgical and anesthesia techniques. The approach is patient- and surgery-specific and involves collaboration and input from multidisciplinary team of health care providers.

CLINICS CARE POINTS

- Orthopedic surgery involving an increased risk of bleeding and need for blood transfusion should incorporate patient and surgery specific blood management strategies.
- Preoperative anemia management is an important step to optimize the patient prior to surgery and physiologically prepare the patient for the surgical stress as well as postoperative course, along with established transfusion guidelines and restrictive hemoglobin triggers.
- Perioperative anticoagulation therapies should be carefully balanced and optimized to reduce the risk of surgical bleeding and thromboembolic events
- Intraoperative blood pressure management, regardless of the anesthetic technique, is an important factor in reducing surgical bleeding and other adverse effects

> • Utilization of tranexamic acid has been shown to significantly decrease surgical bleeding and need for blood transfusion with very favorable patient safety profile.

REFERENCES

1. Yoshihara H, Yoneoka D. National trends in the utilization of blood transfusions in total hip and knee arthroplasty. J Arthroplasty 2014;29(10):1932–7.
2. Slover J, Lavery JA, Schwarzkopf R, et al. Incidence and risk factors for blood transfusion in total joint arthroplasty: analysis of a statewide database. J Arthroplasty 2017;32(9):2684–7.e1.
3. Sizer SC, Cherian JJ, Elmallah RDK, et al. Predicting blood loss in total knee and hip arthroplasty. Orthop Clin North Am 2015;46(4):445–59.
4. Hu SS. Blood loss in adult spinal surgery. Eur Spine J 2004;13(Suppl 1):S3–5.
5. Rawn J. The silent risks of blood transfusion. Curr Opin Anaesthesiol 2008;21(5):664–8.
6. Ponnusamy KE, Kim TJ, Khanuja HS. Perioperative blood transfusions in orthopaedic surgery. J Bone Joint Surg Am 2014;96(21):1836–44.
7. Goel R, Zhu X, Patel EU, et al. Blood transfusion trends in the United States: national inpatient sample, 2015 to 2018. Blood Adv 2021;5(20):4179–84.
8. Lasocki S, Krauspe R, von Heymann C, et al. PREPARE: the prevalence of perioperative anaemia and need for patient blood management in elective orthopaedic surgery: a multicentre, observational study. Eur J Anaesthesiol 2015;32(3):160–7.
9. Gupta PB, DeMario VM, Amin RM, et al. Patient blood management program improves blood use and clinical outcomes in orthopedic surgery. Anesthesiology 2018;129(6):1082–91.
10. Goodnough LT, Shander A. Patient blood management. Anesthesiology 2012;116(6):1367–76.
11. Shander A, Hardy JF, Ozawa S, et al. A global definition of patient blood management. Anesth Analg 2022. https://doi.org/10.1213/ANE.0000000000005873.
12. Althoff FC, Neb H, Herrmann E, et al. Multimodal patient blood management program based on a three-pillar strategy: a systematic review and meta-analysis. Ann Surg 2019;269(5):794–804.
13. Kotzé A, Carter LA, Scally AJ. Effect of a patient blood management programme on preoperative anaemia, transfusion rate, and outcome after primary hip or knee arthroplasty: a quality improvement cycle. Br J Anaesth 2012;108(6):943–52.
14. Muñoz M, Laso-Morales MJ, Gómez-Ramírez S, et al. Pre-operative haemoglobin levels and iron status in a large multicentre cohort of patients undergoing major elective surgery. Anaesthesia 2017;72(7):826–34.
15. Shander A, Knight K, Thurer R, et al. Prevalence and outcomes of anemia in surgery: a systematic review of the literature. Am J Med 2004;116(Suppl 7A):58S–69S.
16. Saleh E, McClelland DBL, Hay A, et al. Prevalence of anaemia before major joint arthroplasty and the potential impact of preoperative investigation and correction on perioperative blood transfusions. Br J Anaesth 2007;99(6):801–8.
17. Fowler AJ, Ahmad T, Phull MK, et al. Meta-analysis of the association between preoperative anaemia and mortality after surgery. Br J Surg 2015;102(11):1314–24.

18. Musallam KM, Tamim HM, Richards T, et al. Preoperative anaemia and postoperative outcomes in non-cardiac surgery: a retrospective cohort study. Lancet 2011;378(9800):1396–407.

19. Smilowitz NR, Oberweis BS, Nukala S, et al. Association between anemia, bleeding, and transfusion with long-term mortality following noncardiac surgery. Am J Med 2016;129(3):315–23.e2.

20. Vaglio S, Prisco D, Biancofiore G, et al. Recommendations for the implementation of a Patient Blood Management programme. Application to elective major orthopaedic surgery in adults. Blood Transfus 2016;14(1):23–65.

21. Goodnough LT, Maniatis A, Earnshaw P, et al. Detection, evaluation, and management of preoperative anaemia in the elective orthopaedic surgical patient: NATA guidelines. Br J Anaesth 2011;106(1):13–22.

22. Mueller MM, Van Remoortel H, Meybohm P, et al. Patient blood management: recommendations from the 2018 frankfurt consensus conference. JAMA 2019; 321(10):983–97.

23. Warner MA, Shore-Lesserson L, Shander A, et al. Perioperative anemia: prevention, diagnosis, and management throughout the spectrum of perioperative care. Anesth Analg 2020;130(5):1364–80.

24. Muñoz M, Acheson AG, Auerbach M, et al. International consensus statement on the peri-operative management of anaemia and iron deficiency. Anaesthesia 2017;72(2):233–47.

25. Camaschella C. Iron deficiency. Blood 2019;133(1):30–9.

26. Hébert PC, Wells G, Blajchman MA, et al. A multicenter, randomized, controlled clinical trial of transfusion requirements in critical care. Transfusion Requirements in Critical Care Investigators, Canadian Critical Care Trials Group. N Engl J Med 1999;340(6):409–17.

27. Carson JL, Hill S, Carless P, et al. Transfusion triggers: a systematic review of the literature. Transfus Med Rev 2002;16(3):187–99.

28. Carson JL, Guyatt G, Heddle NM, et al. Clinical practice guidelines from the AABB: red blood cell transfusion thresholds and storage. JAMA 2016;316(19): 2025–35.

29. Carson JL, Stanworth SJ, Alexander JH, et al. Clinical trials evaluating red blood cell transfusion thresholds: an updated systematic review and with additional focus on patients with cardiovascular disease. Am Heart J 2018;200:96–101.

30. Trentino KM, Farmer SL, Leahy MF, et al. Systematic reviews and meta-analyses comparing mortality in restrictive and liberal haemoglobin thresholds for red cell transfusion: an overview of systematic reviews. BMC Med 2020;18(1):154.

31. Slappendel R, Dirksen R, Weber EWG, et al. An algorithm to reduce allogenic red blood cell transfusions for major orthopedic surgery. Acta Orthop Scand 2003;74(5):569–75.

32. Vassallo R, Goldman M, Germain M, et al, BEST Collaborative. Preoperative autologous blood donation: waning indications in an era of improved blood safety. Transfus Med Rev 2015;29(4):268–75.

33. Forgie MA, Wells PS, Laupacis A, et al. Preoperative autologous donation decreases allogeneic transfusion but increases exposure to all red blood cell transfusion: results of a meta- analysis. Arch Intern Med 1998;158(6):610–6.

34. Etchason J, Petz L, Keeler E, et al. The cost effectiveness of preoperative autologous blood donations. New Engl J Med 1995;332(11):719–24.

35. Billote DB, Glisson SN, Green D, et al. A prospective, randomized study of preoperative autologous donation for hip replacement surgery. JBJS 2002;84(8): 1299–304.

36. Jakovina Blazekovic S, Bicanic G, Hrabac P, et al. Pre-operative autologous blood donation versus no blood donation in total knee arthroplasty: a prospective randomised trial. Int Orthop 2014;38(2):341–6.

37. Kim S, Altneu E, Bou Monsef J, et al. Nonanemic patients do not benefit from autologous blood donation before total knee replacement. HSS J 2011;7(2): 141–4.

38. Devereaux PJ, Mrkobrada M, Sessler DI, et al. Aspirin in patients undergoing noncardiac surgery. N Engl J Med 2014;370(16):1494–503.

39. Levine GN, Bates ER, Bittl JA, et al. 2016 ACC/AHA Guideline Focused Update on Duration of Dual Antiplatelet Therapy in Patients With Coronary Artery Disease: A Report of the American College of Cardiology/American Heart Association Task Force on Clinical Practice Guidelines: An Update of the 2011 ACCF/AHA/SCAI Guideline for Percutaneous Coronary Intervention, 2011 ACCF/AHA Guideline for Coronary Artery Bypass Graft Surgery, 2012 ACC/AHA/ACP/AATS/PCNA/SCAI/STS Guideline for the Diagnosis and Management of Patients With Stable Ischemic Heart Disease, 2013 ACCF/AHA Guideline for the Management of ST-Elevation Myocardial Infarction, 2014 AHA/ACC Guideline for the Management of Patients With Non–ST-Elevation Acute Coronary Syndromes, and 2014 ACC/AHA Guideline on Perioperative Cardiovascular Evaluation and Management of Patients Undergoing Noncardiac Surgery. Circulation 2016; 134(10):e123–55.

40. Horlocker TT, Vandermeuelen E, Kopp SL, et al. Regional anesthesia in the patient receiving antithrombotic or thrombolytic therapy: American Society of Regional Anesthesia and Pain Medicine Evidence-based Guidelines (Fourth Edition). Reg Anesth Pain Med 2018;43(3):263–309.

41. Memtsoudis SG, Cozowicz C, Bekeris J, et al. Anaesthetic care of patients undergoing primary hip and knee arthroplasty: consensus recommendations from the International Consensus on Anaesthesia-Related Outcomes after Surgery group (ICAROS) based on a systematic review and meta-analysis. Br J Anaesth 2019;123(3):269–87.

42. Mauermann WJ, Shilling AM, Zuo Z. A comparison of neuraxial block versus general anesthesia for elective total hip replacement: a meta-analysis. Anesth Analg 2006;103(4):1018.

43. Guay J. The effect of neuraxial blocks on surgical blood loss and blood transfusion requirements: a meta-analysis. J Clin Anesth 2006;18(2):124–8.

44. Wei C, Gu A, Muthiah A, et al. Neuraxial anaesthesia is associated with improved outcomes and reduced postoperative complications in patients undergoing aseptic revision total hip arthroplasty. Hip Int 2020. https://doi.org/10.1177/1120700020975749.

45. Yap E, Wei J, Webb C, et al. Neuraxial and general anesthesia for outpatient total joint arthroplasty result in similarly low rates of major perioperative complications: a multicentered cohort study. Reg Anesth Pain Med 2022. https://doi.org/10.1136/rapm-2021-103189. rapm-2021-103189.

46. Álvarez NER, Ledesma RJG, Hamaji A, et al. Continuous femoral nerve blockade and single-shot sciatic nerve block promotes better analgesia and lower bleeding for total knee arthroplasty compared to intrathecal morphine: a randomized trial. BMC Anesthesiol 2017;17(1):64.

47. Stevens RD, Van Gessel E, Flory N, et al. Lumbar plexus block reduces pain and blood loss associated with total hip arthroplasty. Anesthesiology 2000;93(1): 115–21.

48. Wang H, Ma L, Yang D, et al. Cervical plexus anesthesia versus general anesthesia for anterior cervical discectomy and fusion surgery: A randomized clinical trial. Medicine (Baltimore) 2017;96(7):e6119.
49. Malik O, Brovman EY, Urman RD. The use of regional or neuraxial anesthesia for below-knee amputations may reduce the need for perioperative blood transfusions. Reg Anesth Pain Med 2018;43(1):25–35.
50. Villatte G, Engels E, Erivan R, et al. Effect of local anaesthetic wound infiltration on acute pain and bleeding after primary total hip arthroplasty: the EDIPO randomised controlled study. Int Orthop 2016;40(11):2255–60.
51. Dragan S, Kulej M, Krawczyk A, et al. Methods of reducing allogeneic blood demand in orthopedic surgery. Ortop Traumatol Rehabil 2012;14(3):199–214.
52. Tagarakis GL, Whitlock RP, Gutsche JT, et al. New frontiers in aortic therapy: focus on deliberate hypotension during thoracic aortic endovascular interventions. J Cardiothorac Vasc Anesth 2014;28(3):843–7.
53. Paul JE, Ling E, Lalonde C, et al. Deliberate hypotension in orthopedic surgery reduces blood loss and transfusion requirements: a meta-analysis of randomized controlled trials. Can J Anaesth 2007;54(10):799–810.
54. Jiang J, Zhou R, Li B, et al. Is deliberate hypotension a safe technique for orthopedic surgery?: a systematic review and meta-analysis of parallel randomized controlled trials. J Orthop Surg Res 2019;14(1):409.
55. Wang HY, Yuan MC, Pei FX, et al. Finding the optimal control level of intraoperative blood pressure in no tourniquet primary total knee arthroplasty combine with tranexamic acid: a retrospective cohort study which supports the enhanced recovery strategy. J Orthop Surg Res 2020;15(1):350.
56. Wanner PM, Wulff DU, Djurdjevic M, et al. Targeting higher intraoperative blood pressures does not reduce adverse cardiovascular events following noncardiac surgery. J Am Coll Cardiol 2021;78(18):1753–64.
57. Gregory A, Stapelfeldt WH, Khanna AK, et al. Intraoperative hypotension is associated with adverse clinical outcomes after noncardiac surgery. Anesth Analg 2021;132(6):1654–65.
58. Wijnberge M, Schenk J, Bulle E, et al. Association of intraoperative hypotension with postoperative morbidity and mortality: systematic review and meta-analysis. BJS Open 2021;5(1):zraa018.
59. Sessler DI, Bloomstone JA, Aronson S, et al. Perioperative Quality Initiative consensus statement on intraoperative blood pressure, risk and outcomes for elective surgery. Br J Anaesth 2019;122(5):563–74.
60. Sessler DI, Short TG. Intraoperative hypotension and complications. J Am Coll Cardiol 2021;78(18):1765–7.
61. Pan P, Song K, Yao Y, et al. The impact of intraoperative hypothermia on blood loss and allogenic blood transfusion in total knee and hip arthroplasty: a retrospective study. Biomed Res Int 2020;2020:1096743.
62. Frisch NB, Pepper AM, Rooney E, et al. Intraoperative hypothermia in total hip and knee arthroplasty. Orthopedics 2017;40(1):56–63.
63. Kander T, Schött U. Effect of hypothermia on haemostasis and bleeding risk: a narrative review. J Int Med Res 2019;47(8):3559–68.
64. Sessler DI. Temperature monitoring and perioperative thermoregulation. Anesthesiology 2008;109(2):318–38.
65. Charles-Lozoya S, Cobos-Aguilar H, Manilla-Muñoz E, et al. Survival at 30 days in elderly patients with hip fracture surgery who were exposed to hypothermia: survival study. Medicine (Baltimore) 2021;100(39):e27339.

66. Goel R, Boissonneault A, Grissom H, et al. Impact of intraoperative hypothermia on transfusion requirements in patients with pelvic and acetabular trauma. J Orthop Trauma 2021;35(12):632–6.
67. Jildeh TR, Okoroha KR, Marshall NE, et al. The effect of intraoperative hypothermia on shoulder arthroplasty. Orthopedics 2018;41(4):e523–8.
68. Tedesco NS, Korpi FP, Pazdernik VK, et al. Relationship between hypothermia and blood loss in adult patients undergoing open lumbar spine surgery. J Am Osteopath Assoc 2014;114(11):828–38.
69. Madrid E, Urrútia G, Roqué i Figuls M, et al. Active body surface warming systems for preventing complications caused by inadvertent perioperative hypothermia in adults. Cochrane Database Syst Rev 2016;4:CD009016.
70. Milam JD, Austin SF, Nihill MR, et al. Use of sufficient hemodilution to prevent coagulopathies following surgical correction of cyanotic heart disease. J Thorac Cardiovasc Surg 1985;89(4):623–9.
71. Murray D. Acute normovolemic hemodilution. Eur Spine J 2004;13(Suppl 1): S72–5.
72. Bansal N, Kaur G, Garg S, et al. Acute normovolemic hemodilution in major orthopedic surgery. J Clin Orthop Trauma 2020;11(Suppl 5):S844–8.
73. Rai S, Verma S, Yadav PK, et al. Utility of acute normovolemic hemodilution in major surgeries in rural area: a prospective comparative study from North India. Anesth Essays Res 2017;11(4):909–12.
74. Li Y, Zhang Y, Fang X. Acute normovolemic hemodilution in combination with tranexamic acid is an effective strategy for blood management in lumbar spinal fusion surgery. J Orthop Surg Res 2022;17(1):71.
75. Carless PA, Henry DA, Moxey AJ, et al. Cell salvage for minimising perioperative allogeneic blood transfusion. Cochrane Database Syst Rev 2010;4:CD001888.
76. Stone N, Sardana V, Missiuna P. Indications and outcomes of cell saver in adolescent scoliosis correction surgery: a systematic review. Spine (Phila Pa 1976) 2017;42(6):E363–70.
77. van Bodegom-Vos L, Voorn VM, So-Osman C, et al. Cell salvage in hip and knee arthroplasty: a meta-analysis of randomized controlled trials. J Bone Joint Surg Am 2015;97(12):1012–21.
78. So-Osman C, Nelissen RGHH, Koopman-van Gemert AWMM, et al. Patient blood management in elective total hip- and knee-replacement surgery (part 2): a randomized controlled trial on blood salvage as transfusion alternative using a restrictive transfusion policy in patients with a preoperative hemoglobin above 13 g/dl. Anesthesiology 2014;120(4):852–60.
79. Colomina MJ, Contreras L, Guilabert P, et al. Clinical use of tranexamic acid: evidences and controversies. Braz J Anesthesiol 2021. https://doi.org/10.1016/j. bjane.2021.08.022.
80. Poeran J, Rasul R, Suzuki S, et al. Tranexamic acid use and postoperative outcomes in patients undergoing total hip or knee arthroplasty in the United States: retrospective analysis of effectiveness and safety. BMJ 2014;349:g4829.
81. Fillingham YA, Ramkumar DB, Jevsevar DS, et al. Tranexamic acid in total joint arthroplasty: the endorsed clinical practice guides of the American Association of Hip and Knee Surgeons, American Society of Regional Anesthesia and Pain Medicine, American Academy of Orthopaedic Surgeons, Hip Society, and Knee Society. Reg Anesth Pain Med 2019;44(1):7–11.
82. Fillingham YA, Ramkumar DB, Jevsevar DS, et al. The efficacy of tranexamic acid in total hip arthroplasty: a network meta-analysis. J Arthroplasty 2018; 33(10):3083–9.e4.

83. Xu S, Chen JY, Zheng Q, et al. The safest and most efficacious route of tranexamic acid administration in total joint arthroplasty: A systematic review and network meta-analysis. Thromb Res 2019;176:61–6.

84. Franchini M, Mengoli C, Marietta M, et al. Safety of intravenous tranexamic acid in patients undergoing majororthopaedic surgery: a meta-analysis of randomised controlled trials. Blood Transfus 2018;16(1):36–43.

85. Taeuber I, Weibel S, Herrmann E, et al. Association of Intravenous Tranexamic Acid With Thromboembolic Events and Mortality: A Systematic Review, Meta-analysis, and Meta-regression. JAMA Surg 2021;e210884. https://doi.org/10.1001/jamasurg.2021.0884.

86. Fillingham YA, Ramkumar DB, Jevsevar DS, et al. The safety of tranexamic acid in total joint arthroplasty: a direct meta-analysis. J Arthroplasty 2018;33(10):3070–82.e1.

87. Li G, Sun TW, Luo G, et al. Efficacy of antifibrinolytic agents on surgical bleeding and transfusion requirements in spine surgery: a meta-analysis. Eur Spine J 2017;26(1):140–54.

88. Shu HT, Mikula JD, Yu AT, et al. Tranexamic acid use in pelvic and/or acetabular fracture surgery: a systematic review and meta-analysis. J Orthop 2021;28:112–6.

89. Pecold J, Al-Jeabory M, Krupowies M, et al. Tranexamic acid for shoulder arthroplasty: a systematic review and meta-analysis. J Clin Med 2021;11(1):48.

90. Desborough MJ, Oakland K, Brierley C, et al. Desmopressin use for minimising perioperative blood transfusion. Cochrane Database Syst Rev 2017;7:CD001884.

91. Sánchez AR, Sheridan PJ, Kupp LI. Is platelet-rich plasma the perfect enhancement factor? A current review. Int J Oral Maxillofac Implants 2003;18(1):93–103.

92. Everts PA, Overdevest EP, Jakimowicz JJ, et al. The use of autologous platelet-leukocyte gels to enhance the healing process in surgery, a review. Surg Endosc 2007;21(11):2063–8.

93. Bielecki T, Gazdzik TS, Szczepanski T. Benefit of percutaneous injection of autologous platelet-leukocyte-rich gel in patients with delayed union and nonunion. Eur Surg Res 2008;40(3):289–96.

94. Kuang MJ, Han C, Ma JX, et al. The efficacy of intraoperative autologous platelet gel in total knee arthroplasty: a meta-analysis. Int J Surg 2016;36(Pt A):56–65.

95. Ma J, Sun J, Guo W, et al. The effect of platelet-rich plasma on reducing blood loss after total knee arthroplasty: a systematic review and meta-analysis. Medicine (Baltimore) 2017;96(26):e7262.

96. Bostian PA, Ray JJ, Karolcik BA, et al. Thromboelastography is predictive of mortality, blood transfusions, and blood loss in patients with traumatic pelvic fractures: a retrospective cohort study. Eur J Trauma Emerg Surg 2022;48(1):345–50.

97. Ohrt-Nissen S, Bukhari N, Dragsted C, et al. Blood transfusion in the surgical treatment of adolescent idiopathic scoliosis-a single-center experience of patient blood management in 210 cases. Transfusion 2017;57(7):1808–17.

98. Hagedorn JC, Bardes JM, Paris CL, et al. Thromboelastography for the Orthopaedic Surgeon. J Am Acad Orthop Surg 2019;27(14):503–8.

99. Kaaber AB, Jans Ø, Dziegiel MH, et al. Managing patients on direct factor Xa inhibitors with rapid thrombelastography. Scand J Clin Lab Invest 2021;81(8):661–9.

100. Bai CW, Ruan RX, Pan S, et al. Application of thromboelastography in comparing coagulation difference of rivaroxaban and enoxaparin for

thromboprophylaxis after total hip arthroplasty. J Orthop Surg (Hong Kong) 2021;29(3). https://doi.org/10.1177/23094990211042674.

101. Thomas O, Rein H, Strandberg K, et al. Coagulative safety of epidural catheters after major upper gastrointestinal surgery: advanced and routine coagulation analysis in 38 patients. Perioper Med (Lond) 2016;5:28.

102. Liu C, Guan Z, Xu Q, et al. Relation of thromboelastography parameters to conventional coagulation tests used to evaluate the hypercoagulable state of aged fracture patients. Medicine (Baltimore) 2016;95(24):e3934.

103. Lloyd-Donald P, Lee WS, Liu GM, et al. Thromboelastography in elective total hip arthroplasty. World J Orthop 2021;12(8):555–64.

104. You D, Skeith L, Korley R, et al. Identification of hypercoagulability with thrombelastography in patients with hip fracture receiving thromboprophylaxis. Can J Surg 2021;64(3):E324–9.

105. Bosch P, Kenkre TS, Londino JA, et al. Coagulation profile of patients with adolescent idiopathic scoliosis undergoing posterior spinal fusion. J Bone Joint Surg Am 2016;98(20):e88.

106. Zhang XC, Sun MJ, Pan S, et al. Intravenous administration of tranexamic acid in total hip arthroplasty does not change the blood coagulopathy: a prospective thrombelastography analysis. J Orthop Surg (Hong Kong) 2020;28(3). https://doi.org/10.1177/2309499020959516.

107. Cai DF, Fan QH, Zhong HH, et al. The effects of tourniquet use on blood loss in primary total knee arthroplasty for patients with osteoarthritis: a meta-analysis. J Orthop Surg Res 2019;14(1):348.

108. Huang CR, Pan S, Li Z, et al. Tourniquet use in primary total knee arthroplasty is associated with a hypercoagulable status: a prospective thromboelastography trial. Int Orthop 2021;45(12):3091–100.

109. Ahmed I, Chawla A, Underwood M, et al. Tourniquet use for knee replacement surgery. Cochrane Database Syst Rev 2020;12:CD012874.

110. Falck-Ytter Y, Francis CW, Johanson NA, et al. Prevention of VTE in orthopedic surgery patients: antithrombotic Therapy and Prevention of Thrombosis, 9th ed: American College of Chest Physicians Evidence-Based Clinical Practice Guidelines. Chest 2012;141(2 Suppl):e278S–325S.

111. Chan NC, Siegal D, Lauw MN, et al. A systematic review of contemporary trials of anticoagulants in orthopaedic thromboprophylaxis: suggestions for a radical reappraisal. J Thromb Thrombolysis 2015;40(2):231–9.

112. Kahn SR, Shivakumar S. What's new in VTE risk and prevention in orthopedic surgery. Res Pract Thromb Haemost 2020;4(3):366–76.

113. Anderson DR, Morgano GP, Bennett C, et al. American Society of Hematology 2019 guidelines for management of venous thromboembolism: prevention of venous thromboembolism in surgical hospitalized patients. Blood Adv 2019; 3(23):3898–944.

114. Tafur A, Douketis J. Perioperative management of anticoagulant and antiplatelet therapy. Heart 2018;104(17):1461–7.

115. Palmer AJR, Gagné S, Fergusson DA, et al. Blood management for elective orthopaedic surgery. J Bone Joint Surg Am 2020;102(17):1552–64.

Opioid-Sparing Techniques in Orthopedic Anesthesia—One Step to Opioid-Free Anesthesia?

Helene Beloeil, MD, PhD

KEYWORDS

• Opioid-free • Opioid sparing • Orthopedic anesthesia

KEY POINTS

- Opioid-sparing techniques, especially regional anesthesia have long shown their benefits in orthopedic anesthesia.
- Opioid-free anesthesia is an association of drugs and/or techniques allowing the avoidance of intraoperative opioids.
- Opioid-free anesthesia allows a postoperative morphine sparing and postoperative nausea and vomiting reduction in bariatric/abdominal surgery.
- Opioid-free anesthesia is associated with its own adverse effects.
- Evidences for the benefit of opioid-free anesthesia in orthopedic anesthesia are scarce.

INTRODUCTION

Multimodal postoperative analgesia has been the gold standard for more than 25 years.[1] It allows opioid sparing and better outcomes than morphine administered as a sole analgesic agent after surgery. In orthopedic surgery, regional anesthesia/analgesia is, of course, the best technique to reduce or avoid intraoperative and postoperative opioids. Indeed, the blockage of nociceptive afferences is perfectly ensured by regional anesthesia/analgesia and benefits have been long proven in the literature.[2] However, when regional anesthesia is not feasible or when it is not sufficient, intraoperative opioid-sparing techniques can help reduce opioid consumption and therefore opioid-related side effects. These techniques can ultimately lead to opioid-free anesthesia. Opioid sparing and opioid-free anesthesia should not be separated and put in opposition as they are part of the same global strategy toward less opioid-related side effects due to less opioid administration. Opioid-free anesthesia can be defined as an association of drugs and/or techniques allowing the avoidance of intraoperative opioids. The association can combine NMDA antagonists (ketamine, lidocaine, magnesium

Anesthesia and Intensive Care Department, Univ Rennes, Inserm CIC 1414, COSS 1242, CHU Rennes, Rennes Cedex 35000, France
E-mail address: helene.beloeil@chu-rennes.fr

Anesthesiology Clin 40 (2022) 529–536
https://doi.org/10.1016/j.anclin.2022.06.003
1932-2275/22/© 2022 Elsevier Inc. All rights reserved.

anesthesiology.theclinics.com

Abbreviations	
PROSPECT	procedure specific postoperative pain management
NMDA	N-D Methyl aspartate
POFA	Effect of opioid-free anesthesia on postoperative opioid-related adverse events after major or intermediate non-cardiac surgery
NSAID	non-steroid anti-inflammatory drugs

sulfate), sodium channel blockers (local anesthetics), anti-inflammatory drugs (NSAID, dexamethasone) and alpha-2 agonists (dexmetedomidine, clonidine). Of course, for toxicity reasons, all these drugs/techniques will not be administered simultaneously to the same patient. Moreover, all these drugs have documented side effects. Finally, the protocol of opioid-free or sparing anesthesia has to be tailored to the patient and the procedure.[3]

OPIOID-SPARING TECHNIQUES IN ORTHOPEDIC SURGERY

- The benefit of *regional anesthesia* has been long proven in orthopedic surgery! Regional anesthesia is, of course, the best technique to avoid intraoperative and postoperative opioid during orthopedic surgery.
- Intravenous *lidocaine* administered intravenously blocks sodium channels and discharges of peripheral neurons excited by nociceptive stimuli, inhibits NMDA receptors, and has anti-inflammatory properties. All these effects are clinically translated into an analgesic benefit, morphine sparing, a decrease in the length of stay, an earlier resumption of transit, a reduction in the incidence of nausea and vomiting, and a faster postoperative rehabilitation.[4] This has been mainly shown in abdominal surgery. In orthopedic surgery, IV lidocaine reduced pain scores and morphine consumption in spine surgery.[5] However, some studies did not show any benefit of intravenous lidocaine in spine surgery[6] or total hip arthroplasty.[7] Intravenous lidocaine is, therefore, not recommended by the latest PROSPECT guidelines in orthopedic surgery.[8]
- By antagonizing NMDA receptors, *ketamine* prevents postoperative hyperalgesia. Several meta-analyzes have reported a beneficial effect of ketamine on the intensity of postoperative pain, the reduction of opioid consumption preoperatively and post-operatively, and the reduction of chronic pain after surgery.[9] Ketamine is also helpful in reducing intraoperative blood pressure variability.[10] In spine surgery, especially in patients with preoperative pain and opioid consumption, Loftus and colleagues[11] demonstrated morphine-sparing effects of intraoperative ketamine, with decreased pain scores postoperatively and at 6 weeks. Intraoperative ketamine is recommended during spine surgery.[8] For other orthopedic surgeries, evidences are limited.
- *Magnesium sulfate* is a noncompetitive antagonist of NMDA receptors by inhibition of intracellular calcium flow. Evidences are lacking but some studies have shown morphine sparing when magnesium is administered intraoperatively.[12] Moreover, a meta-analysis reported that magnesium significantly reduces intraoperative heart rate variability.[10,13]
- *Anti-inflammatory drugs* (dexamethasone and NSAIDs) are also helpful when avoiding opioids. NSAIDs spare about 50% in morphine, resulting in a reduction in postoperative nausea and vomiting, sedation, and duration of postoperative ileus, as well as an improvement in pain scores compared with morphine alone. Morphine sparing effect of NSAIDs is more important than the one of paracetamol and nefopam.[14] With regard to dexamethasone, there are now numerous studies

showing morphine savings associated with a reduction in postoperative nausea and vomiting and fatigue and better postoperative rehabilitation with the doses recommended for the prevention of nausea and vomiting; that is, 8 mg. The single dose administered at the beginning of the procedure (0.1 mg/kg) thus allows both a prevention of postoperative nausea and vomiting and an analgesic benefit.[15]

DRUGS ENSURING HEMODYNAMIC STABILITY

Opioids have been used because they provide a good hemodynamic stability. It has been shown several times that intraoperative hemodynamic instability is associated with increased postoperative morbidity. Therefore, as P Forget stated,[10] any strategy oriented to reduce the use of opioids should also minimize the sympathetic response triggered by surgery. Alpha-2 agonists (clonidine, dexmedetomidine) have been proposed to ensure this stability. They allow a direct sympathetic blockade. Due to their pharmacologic characteristics (sedation, hypnosis, anxiolysis, sympatholysis, and analgesia), they are interesting adjuvants to multimodal analgesia/anesthesia. Their antinociceptive effects are attributed to the stimulation of alpha-2 adrenergic receptors located in the central nervous system. The analgesic, antiemetic, and anxiolytic properties of clonidine are well known.[16,17] Dexmedetomidine is more selective agonist of alpha-2 receptors. Its delay of action (6 minutes) and its half-life (2 hours) are shorter than those of clonidine. In terms of side effects, both drugs are associated with risks of hypotension and bradycardia.[18] Meta-analysis have shown that clonidine and dexmedetomidine induce morphine sparing, analgesia and postoperative nausea and vomiting reduction.[19,20] Some studies have chosen to study opioid-free anesthesia with dexmedetomidine with the objective of hemodynamic stability and controlled hypotension.[21,22] Although some studies were negative,[23] most studies reported a good hemodynamic stability with often bradycardia and hypotension with dexmedetomidine (which were the objectives in these studies).[24,25]

Beta blockers have also been proposed to ensure hemodynamic stability during opioid-free anesthesia.[26,27] Studies and meta-analysis have reported benefits in reducing intraoperative and postoperative opioids and postoperative nausea and vomiting. However, the literature is scarce on the subject (β-blockers used during an opioid-free anesthesia) and perioperative administration of β-blockers is associated with specific side effects including a doubt in increasing the risk of stroke.[28]

SOLELY OPIOID-FREE ANESTHESIA IN ORTHOPEDIC SURGERY. WHAT ARE THE BENEFITS?

None of the drugs introduced before allows by one-self performing anesthesia without opioids. However, their association with modern techniques of anesthesia and surgery is an alternative to the use of opioids. Most previous studies on opioid-free anesthesia focused on bariatric and abdominal surgery[29,30] and reported morphine sparing, better recovery, and reduction of postoperative nausea and vomiting. Indeed, Ziemann-Gimmel and colleagues[31] demonstrated a 17% reduction in the risk of postoperative nausea and vomiting by comparing intravenous anesthesia combining propofol-dexmedetomidine-ketamine with an inhaled anesthesia with opioids. Most of the patients included in the POFA study were scheduled for abdominal surgery.[32] This study reported morphine sparing and postoperative nausea and vomiting reduction associated with more opioid-related adverse effects (hypoxemia, sedation) in the patients receiving an opioid-free anesthesia regimen compared with patients receiving an opioid-based anesthesia regimen. Meta-analysis have also reported benefits with opioid-free anesthesia; that is, mostly opioid sparing.[33,34]

The literature is scarce on the potential benefits of opioid-free anesthesia in orthopedic surgery. Studies reporting a benefit of opioid-free anesthesia are either observational,[35] retrospective,[36] or randomized controlled trials with methodological flaws.[37] Indeed, in an observational study on patients scheduled for total hip arthroplasty, opioid-free anesthesia including dexmedetomidine allowed a reduction of postoperative opioid consumption, pain scores, and length of stay when compared with an opioid-based anesthesia regimen including sufentanil.[35] Jolissaint and colleagues[37] reported that opioid-free perioperative management is safe and offers superior pain relief than an opioid management for shoulder arthroplasty. However, the safety of the opioid-free protocol was not studied in this trial, the opioid-free protocol dangerously accumulated local anesthetics vis different routes (nerve block and intravenous lidocaine and bupivacaine infiltration), the detailed intraoperative protocol and opioid consumption are not available, and finally, the opioid-based protocol included only opioid and acetaminophen, postoperatively, which does not follow guidelines on multimodal analgesia. In a retrospective study including only 36 patients who had benefited of spine surgery, total perioperative opioid consumption was reduced by more than 90% with the opioid-free protocol compare with the opioid-based protocol and pain scores were similar.[36]

ARE THERE SPECIFIC INDICATIONS FOR OPIOID-FREE ANESTHESIA?

Patients who can benefit from opioid-free anesthesia are those who are most sensitive to deleterious side effects of opioids. Obese patients and patients suffering from respiratory insufficiency are, of course, crossing mind first. Thus, part of the studies showing the interest of opioid-free anesthesia was performed in obese patients.[38] Other studies are obviously needed to evaluate the real benefit of opioid-free anesthesia in these patients. It can also be assumed that opioid-free anesthesia would be beneficial in patients with respiratory insufficiency or obstructive bronchopneumopathy. However, there is a lack of evidences to validate these indications. Finally, patients suffering from chronic pain and/or consuming opioids before surgery, would be another subpopulation that could benefit the most from opioid-free anesthesia. These patients are at higher risk of severe postoperative acute pain while consuming more postoperative opioids.[39] They have an increased risk of postsurgical pain chronicization.[39] One could hypothesize that reducing opioid-induced hyperalgesia by avoiding intraoperative opioids could reduce postoperative acute and chronic pain and opioid needs in these patients. However, no data are currently available to confirm this hypothesis.

UNANSWERED QUESTIONS AND FUTURE RESEARCH AGENDA

Opioid-free anesthesia is a multimodal anesthesia and therefore consists of a combination of multiple drugs. Many institutions have their own "recipe."[40] However, as presented above, the proofs of the benefits of such combinations of multiple drugs are still scarce in the literature.[41] "Recipes" published without any evidence-based proof of a positive balance of benefits over risks should not be recommended.[42,43] Moreover, the doses of each of the drugs are also not clearly defined because they vary from one study to another. Adverse events have been described with the drugs used to replace opioids,[32] highlighting the critical need for carefully assessing the safety of opioid-free regimens in addition to potential benefit.[43] There is also a need to develop accurate monitoring of intraoperative nociception that is validated during opioid-free anesthesia.[44] Most publications on opioid-free anesthesia involved patients undergoing bariatric surgery. There is a lack of studies showing benefits in other types of surgery, especially orthopedic surgery. Procedure-specific studies are needed. Finally, and most importantly, opioid sparing with multimodal anesthesia/ analgesia regimen has been long proven to benefit the surgical patients. However, opioid sparing is not opioid absence. What are the benefits of an opioid-free anesthesia regimen when compare with an already opioid-sparing regimen? The POFA study showed that the benefit of opioid-free balanced anesthesia is not as outstanding when compared with intraoperative opioids and raises questions about the benefit of eliminating intraoperative opioids when an opioid-sparing regimen is already used.[32]

SUMMARY

Opioid-free anesthesia has been presented as a new paradigm that is revolutionizing our practices. Although multimodal anesthesia and multimodal analgesia have shown undoubtable benefits, studies and data are lacking. Opioid-free anesthesia has never been studied with modern monitoring of intraoperative analgesia. Evidence-based proofs of short-term and long-term benefits as well as procedure-specific documented intraoperative protocols are still yet to come.

DISCLOSURE

The author has nothing to disclose.

REFERENCES

1. Dahl JB, Rosenberg J, Dirkes WE, et al. Prevention of postoperative pain by balanced analgesia. Br J Anaesth 1990;64:518–20.
2. Albrecht E, Chin KJ. Advances in regional anaesthesia and acute pain management: a narrative review. Anaesthesia 2020;75(Suppl 1):e101–10.
3. Shanthanna H, Ladha KS, Kehlet H, et al. Perioperative Opioid Administration: A Critical Review of Opioid-free versus Opioid-sparing Approaches. Anesthesiology 2020. https://doi.org/10.1097/ALN.0000000000003572.
4. Sun Y, Li T, Wang N, et al. Perioperative systemic lidocaine for postoperative analgesia and recovery after abdominal surgery: a meta-analysis of randomized controlled trials. Dis Colon Rectum 2012;55:1183–94.
5. Ibrahim A, Aly M, Farrag W. Effect of intravenous lidocaine infusion on long-term postoperative pain after spinal fusion surgery. Medicine (Baltimore) 2018;97: e0229.
6. Dewinter G, Moens P, Fieuws S, et al. Systemic lidocaine fails to improve postoperative morphine consumption, postoperative recovery and quality of life in patients undergoing posterior spinal arthrodesis. A double-blind, randomized, placebo-controlled trial. Br J Anaesth 2017;118:576–85.
7. Martin F, Cherif K, Gentili ME, et al. Lack of impact of intravenous lidocaine on analgesia, functional recovery, and nociceptive pain threshold after total hip arthroplasty. Anesthesiology 2008;109:118–23.
8. Waelkens P, Alsabbagh E, Sauter A, et al. PROSPECT Working group** of the European Society of Regional Anaesthesia and Pain therapy (ESRA): Pain management after complex spine surgery: A systematic review and procedure-specific postoperative pain management recommendations. Eur J Anaesthesiol 2021; 38:985–94.
9. Brinck EC, Tiippana E, Heesen M, et al. Perioperative intravenous ketamine for acute postoperative pain in adults. Cochrane Database Syst Rev 2018;12: CD012033.

10. Forget P, Cata J. Stable anesthesia with alternative to opioids: Are ketamine and magnesium helpful in stabilizing hemodynamics during surgery? A systematic review and meta-analyses of randomized controlled trials. Best Pract Res Clin Anaesthesiol 2017;31:523–31.

11. Loftus RW, Yeager MP, Clark JA, et al. Intraoperative ketamine reduces perioperative opiate consumption in opiate-dependent patients with chronic back pain undergoing back surgery. Anesthesiology 2010;113:639–46.

12. Murphy JD, Paskaradevan J, Eisler LL, et al. Analgesic efficacy of continuous intravenous magnesium infusion as an adjuvant to morphine for postoperative analgesia: a systematic review and meta-analysis. Middle East J Anaesthesiol 2013;22:11–20.

13. Mahmoud G, Sayed E, Eskander A, et al. Effect of intraoperative magnesium intravenous infusion on the hemodynamic changes associated with right lobe living donor hepatotomy under transesophageal Doppler monitoring-randomized controlled trial. Saudi J Anaesth 2016;10:132–7.

14. Martinez V, Beloeil H, Marret E, et al. Non-opioid analgesics in adults after major surgery: systematic review with network meta-analysis of randomized trials. Br J Anaesth 2017;118:22–31.

15. De Oliveira GS, Almeida MD, Benzon HT, et al. Perioperative single dose systemic dexamethasone for postoperative pain: a meta-analysis of randomized controlled trials. Anesthesiology 2011;115:575–88.

16. De Kock M, Lavandhomme P, Scholtes JL. Intraoperative and postoperative analgesia using intravenous opioid, clonidine and lignocaine. Anaesth Intensive Care 1994;22:15–21.

17. Sanchez Munoz MC, De Kock M, Forget P. What is the place of clonidine in anesthesia? Systematic review and meta-analyses of randomized controlled trials. J Clin Anesth 2017;38:140–53.

18. Demiri M, Antunes T, Fletcher D, et al. Perioperative adverse events attributed to α2-adrenoceptor agonists in patients not at risk of cardiovascular events: systematic review and meta-analysis. Br J Anaesth 2019. https://doi.org/10.1016/j.bja.2019.07.029.

19. Blaudszun G, Lysakowski C, Elia N, et al. Effect of perioperative systemic α2 agonists on postoperative morphine consumption and pain intensity: systematic review and meta-analysis of randomized controlled trials. Anesthesiology 2012;116:1312–22.

20. Schnabel A, Meyer-Frießem CH, Reichl SU, et al. Is intraoperative dexmedetomidine a new option for postoperative pain treatment? A meta-analysis of randomized controlled trials. Pain 2013;154:1140–9.

21. Abdel Hamid MHE. Intravenous Dexmedetomidine Infusion Compared with that of Fentanyl in Patients Undergoing Arthroscopic Shoulder Surgery under General Anesthesia. Anesth Essays Res 2017;11:1070–4.

22. Neil L, Patel A. Effect of Dexmedetomidine Versus Fentanyl on Haemodynamic Response to Patients Undergoing Elective Laparoscopic Surgery: A Double Blinded Randomized Controlled Study. J Clin Diagn Res 2017;11:UC01–4.

23. Lee J, Kim Y, Park C, et al. Comparison between dexmedetomidine and remifentanil for controlled hypotension and recovery in endoscopic sinus surgery. Ann Otol Rhinol Laryngol 2013;122:421–6.

24. Goyal S, Gupta KK, Mahajan V. A Comparative Evaluation of Intravenous Dexmedetomidine and Fentanyl in Breast Cancer Surgery: A Prospective, Randomized, and Controlled Trial. Anesth Essays Res 2017;11:611–6.

25. Vaswani JP, Debata D, Vyas V, et al. Comparative Study of the Effect of Dexmedetomidine Vs. Fentanyl on Haemodynamic Response in Patients Undergoing Elective Laparoscopic Surgery. J Clin Diagn Res 2017;11:UC04–8.
26. Collard V, Mistraletti G, Taqi A, et al. Intraoperative esmolol infusion in the absence of opioids spares postoperative fentanyl in patients undergoing ambulatory laparoscopic cholecystectomy. Anesth Analg 2007;105:1255–62, table of contents.
27. Gelineau AM, King MR, Ladha KS, et al. Intraoperative Esmolol as an Adjunct for Perioperative Opioid and Postoperative Pain Reduction: A Systematic Review, Meta-analysis, and Meta-regression. Anesth Analg 2018;126:1035–49.
28. Study Group POISE, Devereaux PJ, Yang H, et al. Effects of extended-release metoprolol succinate in patients undergoing non-cardiac surgery (POISE trial): a randomised controlled trial. Lancet 2008;371:1839–47.
29. Feld JM, Hoffman WE, Stechert MM, et al. Fentanyl or dexmedetomidine combined with desflurane for bariatric surgery. J Clin Anesth 2006;18:24–8.
30. Mulier JP, Wouters R, Dillemans B, et al. A randomized controlled, double-blind trial evaluating the effect of opioid-free versus opioid general anaesthesia on postoperative pain and discomfort measured bu the QoR-40. J Clin Anesth Pain Med 2018;2:015.
31. Ziemann-Gimmel P, Goldfarb AA, Koppman J, et al. Opioid-free total intravenous anaesthesia reduces postoperative nausea and vomiting in bariatric surgery beyond triple prophylaxis. Br J Anaesth 2014;112:906–11.
32. Beloeil H, Garot M, Lebuffe G, et al. Balanced Opioid-free Anesthesia with Dexmedetomidine versus Balanced Anesthesia with Remifentanil for Major or Intermediate Noncardiac Surgery. Anesthesiology 2021;134:541–51.
33. Olausson A, Svensson CJ, Andréll P, et al. Total opioid-free general anaesthesia can improve postoperative outcomes after surgery, without evidence of adverse effects on patient safety and pain management: A systematic review and meta-analysis. Acta Anaesthesiol Scand 2022;66:170–85.
34. Salomé A, Harkouk H, Fletcher D, et al. Opioid-Free Anesthesia Benefit-Risk Balance: A Systematic Review and Meta-Analysis of Randomized Controlled Trials. J Clin Med 2021;10:2069.
35. Urvoy B, Aveline C, Belot N, et al. Opioid-free anaesthesia for anterior total hip replacement under general anaesthesia: the Observational Prospective Study of Opiate-free Anesthesia for Anterior Total Hip Replacement trial. Br J Anaesth 2021;126:e136–9.
36. Soffin EM, Wetmore DS, Beckman JD, et al. Opioid-free anesthesia within an enhanced recovery after surgery pathway for minimally invasive lumbar spine surgery: a retrospective matched cohort study. Neurosurg Focus 2019;46:E8.
37. Jolissaint JE, Scarola GT, Odum SM, et al. Opioid-free shoulder arthroplasty is safe, effective, and predictable compared to a traditional perioperative opiate regimen: a randomized controlled trial of a novel clinical care pathway. J Shoulder Elbow Surg 2022. https://doi.org/10.1016/j.jse.2021.12.015. S1058-2746(22)00128-8.
38. Singh PM, Panwar R, Borle A, et al. Perioperative analgesic profile of dexmedetomidine infusions in morbidly obese undergoing bariatric surgery: a meta-analysis and trial sequential analysis. Surg Obes Relat Dis 2017;13:1434–46.
39. Montes A, Roca G, Sabate S, et al, GENDOLCAT Study Group. Genetic and Clinical Factors Associated with Chronic Postsurgical Pain after Hernia Repair, Hysterectomy, and Thoracotomy: A Two-year Multicenter Cohort Study. Anesthesiology 2015;122:1123–41.

40. Mauermann E, Ruppen W, Bandschapp O. Different protocols used today to achieve total opioid-free general anesthesia without locoregional blocks. Best Pract Res Clin Anaesthesiol 2017;31:533–45.

41. Lirk P, Rathmell JP. Opioid-free anaesthesia: Con: it is too early to adopt opioid-free anaesthesia today. Eur J Anaesthesiol 2019;36:250–4.

42. Shanthanna H, Ladha KS, Kehlet H, et al. Perioperative Opioid Administration. Anesthesiology 2021;134:645–59.

43. Kharasch ED, Clark JD. Opioid-free Anesthesia: Time to Regain Our Balance. Anesthesiology 2021;134:509–14.

44. Lavand'homme P. Opioid-free anaesthesia: Pro: damned if you don't use opioids during surgery. Eur J Anaesthesiol 2019;36:247–9.

Same Day Joint Replacement Surgery

Patient Selection and Perioperative Management

Catherine Vandepitte, MD, PhD[a], Letitia Van Pachtenbeke, MD[b],
Imré Van Herreweghe, MD[c], Rajnish K. Gupta, MD[d],
Nabil M. Elkassabany, MD, MSCE[e],*

KEYWORDS

- Knee replacement • Knee arthroplasty • Hip replacement • Hip arthroplasty
- Outpatient surgery • Ambulatory surgery • Patient selection

KEY POINTS

- Joint Arthroplasty is shifting from the inpatient setting to same-day ambulatory surgery.
- This shift requires the adaptation of risk stratification, patient selection, and a tailored approach to anesthetic and perioperative management.
- Reported rates of complications after outpatient arthroplasty are comparable to complications in the inpatient settings.
- A tailored perioperative care pathway for outpatient joint arthroplasty patients, taking into account possible local resources, is the key ingredient for success.

INTRODUCTION

Total joint arthroplasty (TJA) is a common surgical procedure, which is anticipated to increase in frequency with the projected increase in life expectancy. The United States Center for Medicare and Medicaid Services (CMS) removed total knee arthroplasty (TKA) in 2018[1] and total hip arthroplasty (THA) in 2020 from the "Inpatient-Only" procedure list. With this change, there is projected to be a tremendous shift of these

[a] Department of Anesthesiology, Ziekenhuis Oost-Limburg, Schiepse Bos 6, Genk 3600, Belgium; [b] Department of Anesthesiology, Ziekenhuis Oost-Limburg (ZOL), Schiepse Bos 6, Genk 3600, Belgium; [c] Department of Anesthesiology, AZ Turnhout, Rubensstraat 166, 2300 Turnhout, Belgium; [d] Department of Anesthesiology, Vanderbilt University Medical Center, 1301 Medical Center Drive 4648, The Vanderbilt Clinic (TVC), Nashville, TN 37232-5614, USA; [e] Department of Anesthesiology and Critical Care, Perelman School of Medicine, University of Pennsylvania, 3400 Spruce Street, Dulles 6, Philadelphia, PA 19104, USA
* Corresponding author.
E-mail address: Nabil.Elkassabany@uphs.upenn.edu
Twitter: @dr_rajgupta (R.K.G.); @nelkassabany (N.M.E.)

Anesthesiology Clin 40 (2022) 537–545
https://doi.org/10.1016/j.anclin.2022.04.003
1932-2275/22/© 2022 Elsevier Inc. All rights reserved.
anesthesiology.theclinics.com

operations from the inpatient setting to same-day ambulatory surgery, whether in the hospital, at hospital-attached ambulatory surgery centers, or at free-standing ambulatory surgery centers. This pivotal change in the traditional inpatient care pattern and reimbursement model requires the adaptation of risk stratification, patient selection, and a tailored approach to anesthetic and perioperative management. The literature on fast-track TJA is scarce with regards to information on strategies to decrease the risk of complications and readmissions when patients are discharged on the same day. The available literature largely focuses on patient selection and pathway design for outpatient joint arthroplasty.[2] Identification of eligible candidates and risk stratification for a same-day total joint replacement is key.[3] The COVID-19 pandemic further emphasized the need for transition from inpatient to ambulatory total joint replacement surgery due to limited hospital bed capacity. In essence, COVID-19 has accelerated a health care model change that was already in progress. The large number of cases that were postponed because of COVID-19 translated into financial losses for the health care industry and impacted patients' health.[3] It was estimated that approximately 30,000 primary and 3000 revision hip and knee arthroplasty procedures would be canceled each week in the United States while COVID-19 restrictions regarding nonessential surgery were in place.[3] The high cancellation rate and the restriction on ward exposure eventually resulted in the conversion of more patients to same-day surgery.[4]

RISK STRATIFICATION TOOLS

A number of scoring systems and assessments tools have been introduced to identify patients who may be eligible for same-day discharge. Age, sex, American Society of Anesthesiologists (ASA) score, body mass index (BMI), obstructive sleep apnea (OSA), malnutrition, chronic opioid use, type of procedure, and comorbidities are ubiquitously present in these studies.[5] Outcome variables that guide these selection criteria are often based on functional capacity, readmissions, reoperations, emergency department visits, urgent unplanned clinic visits, as well as complications.

The "Outpatient Arthroplasty Risk Assessment" (OARA[2]) score is a proprietary scoring system that was designed for the selection of patients ready for same-day and next-day discharge after surgery. The scoring system is based on multi-system analysis of 9 comorbidity areas and scores between 0 and 79 have been found to have more predictive value than the ASA score or the Charlson Comorbidity Index (CCI) for early discharge after TJA. This scoring system has been validated in shoulder and lower limb arthroplasty.[6]

The Risk Assessment and Prediction Tool (RAPT) is another scoring system that does not specifically focus on same-day discharge but rather on discharge disposition and length of stay. It has been validated and it may also be helpful to guide early discharge as it seems to be accurate in low-risk patients.[7] A cohort study[8] by Moore and colleagues assessed the utility of the RAPT score and concluded that it can be used but may be suboptimal for same-day patient discharge when compared with the institutional variables they selected. These variables included BMI and the number of allergies.

COMPLICATION RATES AND BARRIERS FOR SAME-DAY DISCHARGE

The available literature varies in the reporting of complications. Some authors report only readmission rates due to complications,[9,10] whereas others focus on overall surgical or medical complications.[11] Preoperative inclusion criteria may also influence complication rates.[8] This inconsistency in the literature with a large variety of subgroups and different patient selection criteria between studies makes the interpretation of success and complication rates challenging. This leads to the wide range of published complication rates for outpatient TJA.

Analysis of 49,136 patients with TKA of the Medicare database[12] revealed lower complication rates for patients that stayed one postoperative day compared with inpatients or patients that were discharged on the day of surgery (2% vs 8% vs 8%, $P < .001$). Analysis of a large private insurance database[13] with 133,342 patients showed a higher likelihood for surgical site infection, joint stiffness requiring manipulation under anesthesia, component failure requiring revision, and postoperative deep venous thrombosis (DVT) in outpatient TKA. On the other hand, an analysis of 34,416 Medicare patients with THA, found lower outpatient complication rates[14] than inpatient complication rates. The analysis of an insurance claims database did not show any change in outcomes such as all-cause revision surgery, periprosthetic joint infection, prosthetic loosening, prosthetic dislocation, and periprosthetic fracture for in- or outpatients 1 year after surgery.[2]

Complications led to 2.6%[15] readmissions in outpatient TKA and 1.6%[16] in outpatient THA. Outpatient TKAs had lower 30-day readmission rates than the inpatient group. Of note, patients at high risk for readmission were more likely to have a dependent functional status, hypertension, chronic obstructive pulmonary disease, and a prolonged operative time. Most of the readmissions were not surgically related (64%), which included thromboembolic and gastrointestinal complications.[1] In outpatient THA, advanced age and bleeding disorders were significant risk factors for 30-day readmission. Most of the readmissions were surgically related (62%) and included wound complications (27%) and periprosthetic fractures (25%).[16] A systematic review found an overall reoperation rate of 1.9%.[11] Overnight hospital stay reduced the readmission rate for patients with the aforementioned risk factors in THA[16] and TKA.[12] A recent large database analysis of the American College of Surgeons National Surgical Quality Improvement Program (ACS-NSQIP) reported a higher occurrence of cardiac and pulmonary events in outpatient TJA. Patients with older age and bleeding disorders were also more likely to be readmitted,[17] warranting careful selection of outpatient TJA. Long-term follow-up of outpatient patients with TJA oppositely did not reveal any increase in 2-year revision rates, and no differences in unplanned office visits or readmissions.[18,19]

In the analysis of 19 studies with 6519 outpatient THA's or TKA's, Jaibaji and colleagues reported that most of the patients (93.4%) were successfully discharged home on the same day of surgery.[11] The most frequent barriers for same-day discharge included nausea or dizziness, inadequate pain control, hypotension, and urinary retention.

Successful same-day discharge was higher in ambulatory centers than hospital-based centers (97.5% vs 81.4%). The 90-day readmission rate in ambulatory centers was 2.7%, while it was 2.2% for hospitals. The 90-day reoperation rate was 1.82% in ambulatory centers and 0.94% for hospitals.[11]

IMPORTANCE OF PATIENT EDUCATION AND SOCIAL SUPPORT

Outpatient arthroplasty requires comprehensive preoperative counseling, education, and follow-up systems. Common modalities for patient education are informative booklets, joint classes, and mobile phone applications.[20,21] Smartphone platforms will likely become more important as an information platform to guide patients through the perioperative period. Importantly, patients with TJA should understand the ambulatory surgery process, the benefits and risks of same-day discharge, and their own role in the overall experience.[1] In order for patients and their families to feel safe and comfortable with early discharge, their expectations should be set realistically through education.[22] The high patient satisfaction[23] in patients who underwent outpatient arthroplasty, however, may be a result of this intense and focused patient targeted counseling. A practitioner should be available for an after-hours telephone consultation, as outpatient arthroplasties result in more after-hours patient calls.[24]

Home support is considered essential by the American Association of Hip and Knee Surgeons. Many studies include home support (family member or professional caregiver) in the immediate postoperative period as a criterion for eligibility for outpatient surgery.[11] The support at 3 instances—preoperative classes, in the preoperative holding area, and during the last physical therapy session—was shown to improve ambulation targets and readiness for discharge.[25]

INTRAOPERATIVE ANESTHETIC MANAGEMENT

Anesthetic management can modify surgical outcomes and time to discharge. Large database studies mostly provided insights into the optimal anesthetic technique, but few prospective randomized controlled trials are available. The International Consensus on Anesthesia-Related Outcomes after Surgery (ICAROS) group favors primary neuraxial anesthesia over general anesthesia for knee and hip arthroplasty, given documented outcome benefits.[26] In retrospect, spinal anesthesia was also the most commonly used anesthetic technique in outpatient TJA.[11] The use of spinal anesthesia was not related to more adverse events[27] in this population. Postoperative urinary retention has been equally present in both neuraxial and general anesthesia.[28] Reduction of intraoperative fluids or targeted fluid administration[29] have been suggested to decrease the risk of postoperative urinary retention. Proper selection of local anesthetic for spinal anesthesia will reduce delayed recovery.[30]

ANALGESIA FOR AMBULATORY JOINT PROCEDURES

A well-designed multimodal analgesic approach is inherent to the success of same-day TJA programs.[11] A combination of oral analgesics with local anesthetic infiltration, peripheral nerve block, and/or ultrasound-guided infiltration analgesia techniques is reported by most studies.[11] For oral analgesics, paracetamol/acetaminophen, nonsteroidal antiinflammatory drugs, a weak or a strong opioid, as well as adjuncts, are typically used.[11]

Regional analgesia techniques may facilitate the management of postoperative pain, with the goal of minimizing opioid consumption and opioid-related side effects. Motor-sparing regional analgesia techniques are specifically valuable for outpatient surgery as they are less likely to interfere with mobilization or early rehabilitation.[31–33]

As an example, for same-day hip arthroplasty, the pericapsular nerve group (PENG) block results in better preservation of the motor function than a femoral or suprainguinal fascia iliaca block, while preserving the same quality of analgesia to the anterior capsule of the hip.[32] Knee arthroplasty is associated with considerable postoperative pain; therefore, peripheral nerve blocks and/or local infiltration techniques are beneficial. For outpatient TJA, a distal regional analgesia technique, such as adductor canal block, distal femoral triangle block, or genicular blocks reduce motor block and may decrease the risk of postoperative falls.[34] These blocks consist of a blockade of the saphenous nerve and/or smaller sensory branches to the anterior compartment of the knee. Extended analgesia of the posterior compartment of the knee can be provided by surgical local infiltration analgesia or an iPACK (interspace between the popliteal artery and capsule of the posterior knee) block.[35] Although not common, local infiltration analgesia may interfere sometimes with same-day discharge by causing motor block by local anesthetic dispersion toward the sciatic nerve.[36]

IN-HOSPITAL PHYSIOTHERAPY VERSUS HOME NURSING AND HOME PHYSIOTHERAPY

Physiotherapy is crucial after lower limb arthroplasty. Mobilization on the same day of surgery[37] significantly increases the probability of earlier discharge when compared to mobilization on the day after surgery. Little data, however, are available for outpatient arthroplasty rehabilitation. Some studies suggest that there are no differences in patient-reported outcomes or function for same-day discharge after anterior hip arthroplasty when compared with patients who stayed overnight.[38] Telerehabilitation programs are becoming a reality and can allow early rehabilitation at home.[39] For instance, Wang and colleagues report[40] similar outcomes for in-person versus self-directed physiotherapy (PT), with high patient satisfaction and lower costs. Adversely, patients included for self-directed PT may need close follow-up to prevent falls or program failure.[41]

DISCUSSION

The transition to same-day discharge after lower limb total joint replacement is driven by the potential of cost reduction, faster rehabilitation, higher patient satisfaction, and the need for reduced reliance on hospital resources. However, same-day TJA necessitates a comprehensive program, careful patient selection, balanced analgesia, and surgery with a well-designed follow-up program. Currently, only about 15%[42] of all lower limb arthroplasties[12] are performed as outpatient surgery. The recent discontinuation of the designation of both TKA and THA from the CMS "inpatient only" list and the pressures surrounding the COVID-19 pandemic are likely to drive the current trend toward same-day TJA.

An astute selection of patients is critical for a successful same-day program of lower extremity TJA. Several scoring systems to guide same-day discharge have been proposed, such as the RAPT and the OARA, however, significant work needs to be conducted to find an optimal and efficient patient selection algorithm. The RAPT focuses on criteria that guide discharge destination and length of stay (LOS) after hip or knee arthroplasty, but has not been designed specifically for same-day discharge. The OARA score is designed for preoperative patient selection and is validated for outpatient shoulder and lower limb arthroplasty.[5] While comorbidities and patient characteristics can be used for selecting patients, the selection criteria are typically based on individual institutions' preferences, and therefore, challenging to standardize.

Focusing on measures that improve early discharge may additionally reduce the overall length of stay.[43] Similar outcomes have been demonstrated by DeMik et al who found the implementation of a fast-track protocol allowed a switch of selected patients scheduled on the inpatient list to the outpatient list. Importantly, this switch did not result in an increase in complications or readmissions.[44] Another study found that by setting up a fast-track protocol it was possible to discharge 15% of the unselected patients with arthroplasty on the day of surgery.[45]

SUMMARY

There is a growing impetus for same-day TJA to meet financial and logistical challenges and increased demand due to the increasing age of the population. This trend has been accelerated by COVID-19 and limited in-hospital capacity. While the critics of this trend raise the questions about safety, the data from the available outcome studies challenge this safety concern. The overall synthesis of the published experience suggests that by optimizing the constellation of patient education, anesthesia, surgical techniques, postoperative analgesia, and physiotherapy, more patients may be included in fast-track protocols and thus meet the criteria for same-day discharge. Optimization of the perioperative protocols and selection guidelines that facilitate accelerated recovery and early rehabilitation is at the core of the success of the same-day TJA programs.

CLINICS CARE POINTS

- Multidisciplinary approach and good planning are essential to start an outpatient joint replacement program.
- Patient selection, education, and setting the realistic expectation for postoperative course are keys to success.
- Barriers to same discharge include: inadequate pain control, nausea, vomiting, urinary retention, orthostatic hypotension, and failure to achieve the designated physical therapy milestones
- Multimodal analgesia and regional anesthesia and analgesia play a pivotal role in ambulatory joint arthroplasty protocols

DISCLOSURE

R.K. Gupta and N.M. Elkassabany have no relevant financial disclosures.

REFERENCES

1. CMS.gov: Total Knee Arthroplasty (TKA) Removal from the Medicare Inpatient-Only (IPO) List and Application of the 2-Midnight Rule. 2019. Available at: https://www.cms.gov/Outreach-and-Education/Medicare-Learning-Network-MLN/MLNMattersArticles/downloads/SE19002.pdf.
2. Bedard NA, Elkins JM, Brown TS. Effect of COVID-19 on Hip and Knee Arthroplasty Surgical Volume in the United States. J Arthroplasty 2020;35:S45–8.
3. Cherry A, Montgomery S, Brillantes J, et al. Converting hip and knee arthroplasty cases to same-day surgery due to COVID-19. Bone Jt Open 2021;2:545–51.
4. Courtney PM, Boniello AJ, Berger RA. Complications following outpatient total joint arthroplasty: an analysis of a national database. J Arthroplasty 2017;32:1426–30.
5. Polisetty TS, Grewal G, Drawbert H, et al. Determining the validity of the outpatient arthroplasty risk assessment (OARA) tool for identifying patients for safe same-day discharge after primary shoulder arthroplasty. J Shoulder Elbow Surg 2021;30:1794–802.
6. Sconza C, Respizzi S, Grappiolo G, et al. The risk assessment and prediction tool (RAPT) after hip and knee replacement: a systematic review. Joints 2019;07:041–5.
7. Moore MG, Brigati DP, Crijns TJ, et al. Enhanced selection of candidates for same-day and outpatient total knee arthroplasty. J Arthroplasty 2020;35:628–32.
8. Berend KR, Lombardi AV, Berend ME, et al. The outpatient total hip arthroplasty: a paradigm change. Bone Jt J 2018;100-B:31–5.

9. Madsen MN, Kirkegaard ML, Laursen M, et al. Low complication rate after same-day total hip arthroplasty: a retrospective, single-center cohort study in 116 procedures. Acta Orthop 2019;90:439–44.

10. Goyal N, Chen AF, Padgett SE, et al. Otto Aufranc Award: A Multicenter, Randomized Study of Outpatient versus Inpatient Total Hip Arthroplasty. Clin Orthop 2017; 475:364–72.

11. Jaibaji M, Volpin A, Haddad FS, et al. Is Outpatient Arthroplasty Safe? A Systematic Review. J Arthroplasty 2020;35:1941–9.

12. Courtney PM, Froimson MI, Meneghini RM, et al. Can total knee arthroplasty be performed safely as an outpatient in the medicare population? J Arthroplasty 2018;33:S28–31.

13. Arshi A, Leong NL, D'Oro A, et al. Outpatient total knee arthroplasty is associated with higher risk of perioperative complications. J Bone Joint Surg 2017;99: 1978–86.

14. Greenky MR, Wang W, Ponzio DY. Courtney PM: Total hip arthroplasty and the medicare inpatient-only list: an analysis of complications in medicare-aged patients undergoing outpatient surgery. J Arthroplasty 2019;34:1250–4.

15. Bovonratwet P, Shen TS, Ast MP, et al. Reasons and Risk factors for 30-day readmission after outpatient total knee arthroplasty: a review of 3015 cases. J Arthroplasty 2020;35:2451–7.

16. Bovonratwet P, Chen AZ, Shen TS, et al. What are the reasons and risk factors for 30-day readmission after outpatient total hip arthroplasty? J Arthroplasty 2021;36: 258–63.e1.

17. AAHKS AA of H and KS: CMS Releases CY2020 OPPS and ASC Payment Systems. Available at: https://www.aahks.org/advocacy/cy2020-opps-asc-pr/.

18. Rosinsky PJ, Chen SL, Yelton MJ, et al. Outpatient vs. inpatient hip arthroplasty: a matched case-control study on a 90-day complication rate and 2-year patient-reported outcomes. J Orthop Surg 2020;15:367.

19. Malahias M-A, Gu A, Richardson SS, et al. Hospital discharge within a day after total hip arthroplasty does not compromise 1-year outcomes compared with rapid discharge: an analysis of an insurance claims database. J Arthroplasty 2020;35: S107–12.

20. European HC: give your hip a new future. Available at: https://heuppraktijk.be/en/#begeleiding.

21. Hip Analysis Center. Available at: https://heuppraktijk.be/en/hip-analysis-centre/.

22. Adelani MA, Barrack RL. Patient perceptions of the safety of outpatient total knee arthroplasty. J Arthroplasty 2019;34:462–4.

23. Hoffmann JD, Kusnezov NA, Dunn JC, et al. The shift to same-day outpatient joint arthroplasty: a systematic review. J Arthroplasty 2018;33:1265–74.

24. Shah RP, Karas V, Berger RA. Rapid discharge and outpatient total joint arthroplasty introduce a burden of care to the surgeon. J Arthroplasty 2019;34: 1307–11.

25. Theiss MM, Ellison MW, Tea CG, et al. The connection between strong social support and joint replacement outcomes. Orthopedics 2011;34(5):357.

26. Memtsoudis SG, Cozowicz C, Bekeris J, et al. Anaesthetic care of patients undergoing primary hip and knee arthroplasty: consensus recommendations from the International Consensus on Anaesthesia-Related Outcomes after Surgery group (ICAROS) based on a systematic review and meta-analysis. Br J Anaesth 2019; 123:269–87.

27. Kendall MC, Cohen AD, Principe-Marrero S, et al. Spinal versus general anesthesia for patients undergoing outpatient total knee arthroplasty: a national

propensity-matched analysis of early postoperative outcomes. BMC Anesthesiol 2021;21:226.

28. Ziemba-Davis M, Nielson M, Kraus K, et al. Identifiable risk factors to minimize postoperative urinary retention in modern outpatient rapid recovery total joint arthroplasty. J Arthroplasty 2019;34:S343–7.

29. Mathew M, Ragsdale TD, Pharr ZK, et al. Risk factors for prolonged time to discharge in total hip patients performed in an ambulatory surgery center due to complaints of the inability to void. J Arthroplasty 2021;36:3681–5.

30. Schwenk ES, Kasper VP, Smoker JD, et al. Mepivacaine *versus* bupivacaine spinal anesthesia for early postoperative ambulation. Anesthesiology 2020;133: 801–11.

31. Kwofie MK, Shastri UD, Gadsden JC, et al. The effects of ultrasound-guided adductor canal block versus femoral nerve block on quadriceps strength and fall risk: a blinded, randomized trial of volunteers. Reg Anesth Pain Med 2013; 38:321–5.

32. Aliste J, Layera S, Bravo D, et al. Randomized comparison between pericapsular nerve group (PENG) block and suprainguinal fascia iliaca block for total hip arthroplasty. Reg Anesth Pain Med 2021;46:874–8.

33. Kim DH, Beathe JC, Lin Y, et al. Addition of infiltration between the popliteal artery and the capsule of the posterior knee and adductor canal block to periarticular injection enhances postoperative pain control in total knee arthroplasty: a randomized controlled trial. Anesth Analg 2019;129:526–35.

34. Elkassabany NM, Antosh S, Ahmed M, et al. The risk of falls after total knee arthroplasty with the use of a femoral nerve block versus an adductor canal block: a double-blinded randomized controlled study. Anesth Analg 2016;122: 1696–703.

35. Kandarian B, Indelli PF, Sinha S, et al. Implementation of the IPACK (Infiltration between the Popliteal Artery and Capsule of the Knee) block into a multimodal analgesic pathway for total knee replacement. Korean J Anesthesiology 2019; 72(3):238–44.

36. Keulen MHF, Asselberghs S, Bemelmans YFL, et al. Reasons for unsuccessful same-day discharge following outpatient hip and knee arthroplasty: 5½ years' experience from a single institution. J Arthroplasty 2020;35:2327–34.e1.

37. Okamoto T, Ridley RJ, Edmondston SJ, et al. Day-of-surgery mobilization reduces the length of stay after elective hip arthroplasty. J Arthroplasty 2016;31: 2227–30.

38. Zomar BO, Bryant DM, Hunter SW, et al. Perioperative gait analysis after total hip arthroplasty: Does outpatient surgery compromise patient outcomes? Can J Surg 2021;64:E407–13.

39. Nelson M, Bourke M, Crossley K, et al. Telerehabilitation is non-inferior to usual care following total hip replacement — a randomized controlled non-inferiority trial. Physiotherapy 2020;107:19–27.

40. Wang WL, Rondon AJ, Tan TL, et al. Self-directed home exercises vs outpatient physical therapy after total knee arthroplasty: value and outcomes following a protocol change. J Arthroplasty 2019;34:2388–91.

41. Klement MR, Rondon AJ, McEntee RM, et al. Web-based, self-directed physical therapy after total knee arthroplasty is safe and effective for most, but not all, patients. J Arthroplasty 2019;34:S178–82.

42. Outpatient Joint Replacement: An Unnecessary Concern or Market Reality?. Available at: https://newsroom.vizientinc.com/outpatient-joint-replacement-an-unnecessary-concern-or-market-reality.htm.

43. Morrell AT, Layon DR, Scott MJ, et al. Enhanced recovery after primary total hip and knee arthroplasty: a systematic review. J Bone Jt Surg 2021;103(20): 1938–47.
44. DeMik DE, Carender CN, An Q, et al. Has removal from the inpatient-only list increased complications after outpatient total knee arthroplasty? J Arthroplasty 2021;36:2297–301.e1.
45. Gromov K, Kjærsgaard-Andersen P, Revald P, et al. Feasibility of outpatient total hip and knee arthroplasty in unselected patients: a prospective 2-center study. Acta Orthop 2017;88:516–21.

What Do Orthopedic Trauma Surgeons Want and Expect from Anesthesiologists?

Christian Pean, MD, MS[a], Michael J. Weaver, MD[a],
Mitchel B. Harris, MD[b], Thuan Ly, MD[b],
Arvind G. von Keudell, MD, MPH[a,c,*]

KEYWORDS

- Orthogeriatrics • Fractures • Frailty • Perioperative medicine • Trauma
- Polytrauma • Health systems • Health policy

KEY POINTS

- A multidisciplinary approach is necessary to care for polytrauma patients with airway protection and resuscitation the priorities of the anesthesiologist.
- Orthopedic trauma surgery is often painful for patients and benefits from multimodal pain management including peripheral nerve blocks for appropriate injuries.
- Orthogeriatrics is an emerging field requiring specialized input from geriatricians to aid anesthesiologists in managing perioperative care issues.
- Orthopedic trauma surgeons prioritize timely fixation and closed-loop communication in the process of caring for fracture patients. The input and insight of the treating anesthesiologist early in an orthopedic patient's care is critical.

INTRODUCTION

Trauma is responsible for significant morbidity and mortality worldwide, and in the United States, trauma is the number one cause of death for patients between the ages of 1 and 44.[1] Orthopedic trauma patients present several unique challenges to anesthesiologists. In the acute setting, the priority for polytraumatized patients is immediate cardiopulmonary resuscitation, hemodynamic stabilization, and the acute attention to life-threatening injuries. However, many patients with orthopedic injuries warrant dynamic consideration for the timing of operative intervention.[2] This coordination of care requires thoughtful input from the orthopedic trauma surgeon and

[a] Brigham and Women's Hospital, 75 Francis Street, Boston, MA 02115, USA; [b] Massachusetts General Hospital, 55 Fruit Street #14, Boston, MA 02114, USA; [c] Bispebjerg Hospital, Universtiy of Copenhagen, Bispebjerg Bakke 23, Copenhagen, KBH 2400, Denmark
* Corresponding author.
E-mail address: avonkeudell@bwh.harvard.edu

Anesthesiology Clin 40 (2022) 547–556
https://doi.org/10.1016/j.anclin.2022.06.004
1932-2275/22/© 2022 Elsevier Inc. All rights reserved.

anesthesiologist alike. Data on the benefit of early surgical treatment for patients with femur and hip fractures have been available for decades; however, the frailty and co-morbidity profile of geriatric patients in the United States can make timely medical optimization before surgery difficult. One-year mortality for patients over 75 years of age with hip fractures can exceed 30%, and interdisciplinary communication from the anesthesiologist, consulting geriatric and medical services, and the orthopedic trauma surgeon is critical.[3–7]

Ultimately, optimal management of orthopedic trauma patients requires anesthesiologists and orthopedic trauma surgeons to align their priorities in the best interest of the patient in conjunction with the medical or geriatrics services. Common goals for the orthopedic trauma surgeon and anesthesiologist should include safe, expeditious surgery, and optimal perioperative pain management that permits monitoring for post-traumatic sequelae such as compartment syndrome.[8,9]

In this article, we aim to highlight clinical concepts relevant to orthopedic trauma surgeons and anesthesiologists managing these patients. By focusing on team expectations and system-based approaches to management, orthopedic trauma surgeons and anesthesiologists can rely on the strategies outlined in this article to successfully deliver the highest quality of care to their mutual patients.

POLYTRAUMATIZED PATIENTS: EARLY APPROPRIATE CARE AND DAMAGE CONTROL ORTHOPEDICS

Anesthesiologists are often involved early in the care of multiply injured patients with life-threatening diaphyseal fractures, open fractures, or pelvic and acetabular fractures. Adherence to advanced trauma life support protocols and initial stabilization is critical to early treatment coordination. Airway protection is often compromised in these patients, polytrauma teams led by trauma general surgeons with input from emergency physicians, and subspecialty consultants vary in their protocols between institutions but primarily focus on hemodynamic stability and early resuscitative measures.[10] Establishing a close working relationship between the acute care surgery, orthopedic trauma surgery, and anesthesiology teams is an important component of decision-making for perioperative management in polytrauma patients. Consistent communication between all involved consulting services is paramount to success. The decision for timing of operative intervention must be made in coordinated fashion but ultimately led by the anesthesiologist. It is worth consideration for the acute care surgeons to be communicated with the anesthesiology team and orthopedic trauma surgery teams during intervention and particularly approaching the end of orthopedic intervention (**Fig. 1**). A similar triad of care involving geriatricians is warranted for elderly, medically complex orthogeriatric patients.

General anesthesia with intraoperative monitoring of hemodynamic status is standard for these patients, and the orthopedic trauma perspective often hinges on decisions for temporizing stabilization versus definitive fixation for long bone fractures as well as timely control of pelvic and acetabular hemorrhage.[11–13] Angiographic embolization for patients with pelvic and acetabular fractures in the setting of continued hemodynamic instability should also be carefully planned with the orthopedic trauma surgeon, interventional radiologist, anesthesiologist, and trauma surgery teams.

Although the specific considerations of early appropriate care, early total care, and damage control orthopedics are beyond the scope of this article, it is useful for anesthesiologists and orthopedic trauma surgeons alike to appreciate the fundamental basis of initial fracture stabilization in the polytrauma setting. We adhere to the principles of early appropriate care popularized by Vallier and colleagues.[14] Early appropriate

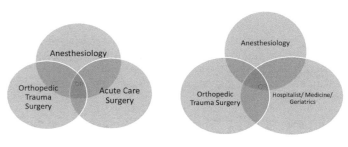

Polytrauma   Elderly/medically complex patients

Fig. 1. Managing polytraumatized and orthogeriatric patients: It is imperative that in the management of polytraumatized patients, there is an understanding of the intricate relationship between the three critical clinical services in patient perioperative management between anesthesiology, orthopedic trauma surgery, and acute care surgeons (*left*). Similarly, orthogeriatric patient management mandates a constant clear flow of communication between the hospitalist/medical team, anesthesiology, and orthopedic trauma surgery teams (*right*). Decisions regarding the patient's stability for initiating or continuing operative management are made together, but ultimately fall to the anesthesiologist. OR, operating room.

care consists of treating the most time-critical orthopedic injuries early with definitive treatment while minimizing the secondary inflammatory response. Studies have indicated that this approach has several benefits including improved postoperative mortality and morbidity and better quality of care outcomes such as decreased length of stay, increased hospital revenues, and decreased delays to surgery. Typical laboratory parameters for proceeding with early appropriate care include a lactate less than 4.0, a base excess greater than -5.5 and pH >7.25. Other useful laboratory values signaling acidosis and adequacy of resuscitation include interleukin (IL)-1, IL-6, IL-8, and IL-10 and tumor necrosis factor-alpha levels.[1,15]

For anesthesiologists in the polytrauma setting, information regarding any blood products the patient has received, shifts in fluid status, the need for postoperative critical care coordination, and signs of intraoperative hemodynamic and metabolic instability should be communicated early and often to the orthopedic trauma surgeon. Similarly the surgeon should be communicating the amount of blood loss encountered and the possible length of any interventions. In unstable patients with pelvic fractures, initial temporizing surgical measures such as external fixation are performed with the intent to improve hemodynamic stability with the patient positioned supine. A systematic approach to communication should be implemented between the orthopedic trauma surgeon and the anesthesiologist regarding critical patient issues such as cardiorespiratory decline, hemodynamic instability, or airway issues. Similarly, orthopedic trauma surgeons are expected to communicate sudden bleeding encountered, challenges of fracture fixation, and estimation of procedure length as the case proceeds. There are often "bail out" options if patients either fail to respond to treatment or become unstable. A good working relationship and early communication of problems encountered on either side of the drapes can aide in providing optimal patient care.

Another nuance of polytrauma orthopedic care is ensuring safe sign outs during transitions of care to postoperative recovery hospital staff or critical care teams. This communication should include the anesthesiologist and a member of the orthopedic team present for the entire sign out. Information regarding pressure requirements, cardiac abnormalities, or respiratory compromise noted intraoperatively by the anesthesiologist may not be noted by the orthopedic trauma surgeon until it is reported during these transitions of care. These handoffs are an opportunity to ensure the appropriate level of care is catered to the patient postoperatively as well as to synchronize perioperative management expectations of the anesthesiologist and orthopedic traumatologist. We have outlined these facets of care coordination and others from initial patient evaluation to discharge for orthopedic trauma surgeons and anesthesiologists to consider in a diagram (**Fig. 2**).

"Is the Patient Cleared for Surgery?": Preoperative Cardiac Evaluation and Risk Optimization

Medical optimization of patients before surgery is an important process of concern for orthopedic trauma surgeons. The euphemism "is the patient cleared for surgery?" encapsulates this sentiment. A common challenge for orthopedic trauma surgeons is disagreement regarding medical optimization between the hospitalist or medical team and the treating anesthesiologist if these services are involved. Avoiding miscommunication between anesthesiologists, medical physicians including geriatricians, and orthopedic trauma surgeons is facilitated by the establishment of guidelines for preoperative risk optimization. In addition to establishing preoperative risk optimization guidelines, it is also important to consider transitions in care between providers as comfort levels to proceed with surgery vary between different anesthesiologists.

Several studies have indicated there is an overreliance on medical testing before surgical procedures.[16–18] Whereas preoperative testing resulting in delays to surgical intervention can be thought of as unnecessary to the orthopedic trauma surgeon, it is useful to review the rationale for some of the more time-consuming preoperative tests such as echocardiography for hip fractures. Any preoperative procedure or laboratory test conducted should be based on the premise that results from the investigation will enable one of the following:

1. Correction of detected abnormalities
2. Quantification of risk for prognostic purposes and setting patient expectations
3. Modification of surgical, anesthetic, or medical management in the interest of the patient's well-being.

Adoption of standardized protocols and algorithms for preoperative risk stratification can counteract proclivities toward unnecessary testing that may not change the acute management of the patient. We suggest these protocols could be established with leadership input from general trauma surgeons, orthopedic trauma surgeons,

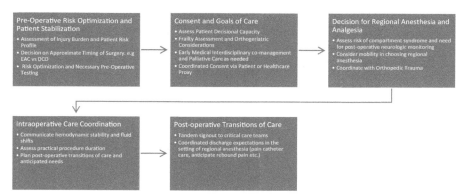

Fig. 2. Orthopedic trauma surgeon and anesthesiologist dyad flow approach to care.

cardiologists, hospitalists/geriatricians, and anesthesiologists at the institution to streamline the care to these patients. In addition to agreeing on testing parameters, critical stakeholders who put processes in place also collect data that track adherence to the agreed on guidelines and identify reasons for straying from established protocols. Regular audits of quality metrics can be beneficial. Tracking trends in time from admission to surgery, postoperative cardiac morbidity, frequency of testing, preoperative testing-related expenditures and frequency of unnecessary laboratory orders can help streamline surgical optimization pathways.

It should also be well established that the decision on whether a patient is clinically stable enough to undergo operative management ultimately lies with the anesthesiologist. It is the responsibility of the orthopedic trauma surgeon to communicate information to the anesthesiologist on expected outcomes of delayed surgery for a given fracture, but always within the context of the patient's resuscitative status. The maxim "life over limb" is well applied in these scenarios. It is critical to foster an environment in which anesthesiologists feel comfortable and confident delaying a surgical case in light of physiologic data or canceling a case outright if it is deemed unsafe to proceed based on their clinical judgment. In the scenario that a case needs to be canceled or delayed, it is good practice for the anesthesiologist to clearly communicate the reasons for cancellation to the involved treatment teams, specifically acute care surgery, hospitalist, and orthopedic surgery teams. Any further studies or resuscitative parameters that would permit surgical intervention in the near future should also be communicated.

ORTHOGERIATRIC PATIENTS

An increasing number of geriatric patients require orthopedic trauma care for injuries such as hip fractures, distal femur fractures, or periprosthetic joint fractures. Several studies have indicated expeditious care for hip fractures has been tied to benefits in morbidity and mortality.[19–22] A baseline expectation should be that orthopedic trauma surgeons and anesthesiologists facilitate the option for surgical intervention for hip fractures within 24 to 48 hours of injury. Although expedient treatment is preferable, it should also be noted that in the recent Hip ATTACK study, a randomized clinical trial comparing accelerated surgery within 6 hours of diagnosis compared with standard of care, there was no difference in risk of mortality or complication with accelerated surgery (within 6 hours of diagnosis).[23]

Guidelines for hip fracture care developed in the United Kingdom also emphasize the early implementation of fascia iliaca blocks for pain control in these patients and outline specific circumstances for delaying hip fracture care in the setting of high medical risk comorbidities.[8] Orthogeriatric guidelines may vary by institution based on care capacity and infrastructure, but agreement on pathways to surgical optimization and establishing quality of care parameters with input from anesthesiologists and orthopedic trauma surgeons will facilitate consistent improved care delivery.

Geriatric care coordination with a hospitalist team for elderly fracture patients confers several benefits and also introduces additional input for preoperative and postoperative management (see **Fig. 1**). This may add a layer of complexity to the interdisciplinary approach of orthopedic surgical care. Ensuring clear alignment of preoperative and postoperative goals of care for elderly orthopedic trauma patients with guarded prognoses is another important facet of care coordination between orthopedic trauma surgeons, hospitalist/geriatricians, and anesthesiologists. The authors previously published an article on a holistic approach to geriatric patient fracture care (**Fig. 3**).[24] We recommend early palliative care involvement for higher

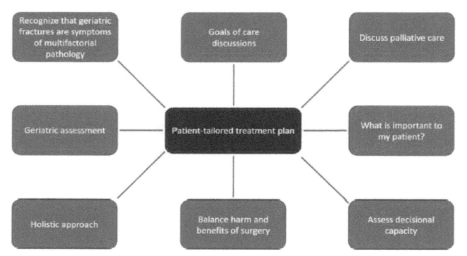

Fig. 3. A holistic approach to geriatric fracture patients. (Reproduced with permission from author AVK.)

risk patients and accounting for the risk of postoperative delirium in decisions for anesthetic and analgesic medications delivered by the anesthesiology team.[25]

Acquisition of consent for surgery and anesthesia should be coordinated, particularly for patients lacking cognitive competency. A proactive consent process that engages the health care proxy of a patient in a single care episode can prevent potential ethical dilemmas and surgical delays.[26] This practice also streamlines communication with the patient's family regarding expectations and risks of surgery. Sometimes it is worth asking "Should we perform surgery?" rather than "Can we perform surgery?" Although most of the patients benefit in terms of pain control, self-care, and the ability to regain ambulatory status, there is a role for palliative care in select patients. The routine assessment of cognitive status not only aids in assessing decision-making capacity but also adds useful information for postoperative care. The Mini-Cog test is derived from the Montreal Cognitive Assessment and has been shown to correlate with a higher risk of complications for geriatric fracture patients.[27] A Mini-Cog assessment of 3 or less suggests cognitive impairment and should be further investigated postoperatively.

REGIONAL ANESTHESIA AND MULTIFACETED PAIN MANAGEMENT COORDINATION

Patients and physicians alike are cognizant of pain burden after acute musculoskeletal injuries. Pain is not only potentially mentally debilitating for patients, but the physiologic impact of severe pain can critically impact mobility and in turn increase risks related to recumbency such as hindered pulmonary toilet, pulmonary embolism, development of ulcers, joint stiffness, and other unfavorable patient outcomes. The opioid crisis in the United States has decimated communities, and the increases in opioid-related deaths and complications have guided nuanced approaches to pain management in the American health care system. Although the US population makes up 5% of the global population, 80% of opioid consumption is estimated to occur in the United States. This social context has accentuated the appeal of regional anesthetic methods and peripheral nerve blocks (PNBs).[28]

In a study by Kandemir and colleagues, a useful color-coded figure outlines general considerations for cases in which regional anesthesia is appropriate as well as

Approach for Preoperative Peripheral Nerve Blocks in Orthopaedic Trauma Surgery

Green	Yellow	Red	Universal Precautions
PNB OK.	Consult surgical attending before PNB. Post-op PNB may be OK after detailed neurologic examination	PNB **NOT** indicated. PNB OK only if approved by surgical attending.	• Appropriate consideration and discussion with the patient regarding the risks and benefits of peripheral nerve block (PNB). • Site marking • Documentation of consent.
Upper Extremity • Distal radius fracture > 48 hrs from injury • Clavicle fractures • Olecranon fractures • Hand fractures • Incision and drainage • Removal of implant	• Proximal humerus fractures • Shoulder fracture dislocations • Humeral shaft fractures • Elbow fractures	• Distal radius fractures <48 hours from fracture • Forearm fractures • Elbow fracture dislocations • Forearm lacerations • Crush injuries	• Detailed neurologic examination and documentation before PNB is done. • Use of nerve block cart with all materials • Safe and sterile procedural technique and documentation (preprocedure time-out with confirmation of correct patient, indication, and side; appropriate patient monitoring ; use of real-time ultrasonography guidance with avoidance of needle to nerve contact and vascular puncture; aspiration and injection of appropriately dosed local anesthetic)
Lower Extremity • Hip fractures • Patella fractures • Low-energy ankle fractures • Foot fractures • Incision and drainage • Removal of implant	• Low-energy tibial plateau fractures (Schatzker Types I, II, and III) • Low-energypilon fractures • Ankle fracture dislocations • High-energy ankle fractures • Hindfoot and midfoot fracture dislocations	• Femoral shaft fractures • Tibial shaft fractures • High-energytibial plateau fractures (Schatzker Types IV, V, and VI) • High-energypilon fractures • Osteotomies • Polytrauma • Any injury with evidence of neurovascular injury or clinical concern for compartment syndrome	• Presence of necessary resuscitation equipment and intralipid in case of local anesthetic toxicity reaction. • Detailed neurologic exam and documentation after PNB is performed. • Clear marking of extremity and documentation of PNB details in the medical record. • Verbal communication of PNB details with participating clinical teams • Appropriate post-PNB care of weakened or insensate extremity to prevent limb injury (e.g., falls). • Post-PNB instructions provided.

Fig. 4. Approach to peripheral nerve blocks. (Reproduced with permission from authors.[14])

circumstances for conferring with the orthopedic traumatologist before administering regional anesthesia. Early mobilization of geriatric fracture patients is paramount to improving functional and clinical outcomes in this patient population.[23] To that end, utilization of pain catheters or regional blocks that impede mobility should be discussed in detail with the orthopedic trauma team before being administered (**Fig. 4**). For orthopedic trauma surgeons, a preoperative assessment of limb swelling and nerve function in extremity fractures will inform the appropriateness of regional anesthesia. High-risk injuries for compartment syndrome such as tibial shaft fractures, bicondylar tibial plateau fractures, and high-energy upper extremity injuries may preclude the ability to administer regional anesthesia.

An often encountered issue regarding regional anesthetic blocks is reconciliation of postoperative communication and follow-up between the patient, the anesthesiologist, and the surgeon. Because discharge instructions and follow-up are coordinated by the orthopedic team, information regarding expectations after regional blocks may be overlooked. "Rebound pain," a phenomenon of increased unexpected postoperative pain following the waning effects of a PNB, can be distressing for patients and result in unnecessary emergency department visits or readmissions.[29] Carefully crafted patient discharge information and telehealth or digital information guides can help patients cope with the onset of postoperative pain with a predetermined initiation of oral analgesic medications or other adjunct analgesic methods such as ice, elevation, or medicated patches.

SUMMARY

Coordinating high-quality surgical care for orthopedic trauma patients presents many multifaceted challenges for surgeons and anesthesiologists. However, with a team-based approach and proper infrastructure, orthopedic trauma surgeons and anesthesiologists can implement systems that expedite care, prevent complications, and improve the perioperative experience for patients and physicians alike. Critical components to achieving these goals include fluid communication and setting early expectations and protocols for anticipated orthopedic trauma scenarios. Applying the principles reviewed in this article should aid multidisciplinary orthopedic trauma teams provide the highest quality care for their patients.

CLINICS CARE POINTS

- Avoid peripheral nerve blocks in patients with high-energy long bone fractures at risk for compartment syndrome and consult with the orthopedic traumatologist on periarticular fractures before administering peripheral nerve blocks.

- Medical optimization for polytrauma patients is guided by the "early appropriate care" approach, and laboratory data such as a base deficit greater than −5.5 and a lactate less than 4.0 are evidence-based parameters indicating it is safe to proceed with definitive fixation for some of these injuries.

- Orthogeriatric care benefits from coordinated input from the anesthesiologist, orthopedic surgeon, and a geriatrician to guide medical optimization.

- The decision to proceed with surgery in the setting of orthopedic injury is best made in a closed loop of communication between the primary admitting team, the orthopedic surgeon, and the anesthesiologist with careful consideration of costs and benefits of preoperative tests versus timely operative intervention.

FUNDING

The authors received no financial support for the research, authorship, and/or publication of the article.

DISCLOSURE

None of the authors declared financial, consultant, institutional, or other disclosures related to the research in this article.

REFERENCES

1. Vallier HA, Como JJ, Wagner KG, et al. Team Approach: Timing of Operative Intervention in Multiply-Injured Patients. JBJS Rev 2018;6(8):e2.
2. Han G, Wang Z, Du Q, et al. Damage-control orthopedics versus early total care in the treatment of borderline high-energy pelvic fractures. Orthopedics 2014; 37(12):e1091–100.
3. Sheehan KJ, Sobolev B, Guy P. Mortality by Timing of Hip Fracture Surgery. J Bone Joint Surg Am 2017;99(20):e106.
4. Mehr DR, Tatum PE, Crist BD. Hip Fractures in Patients With Advanced Dementia. JAMA Intern Med 2018;178(6):780.
5. Williamson S, Landeiro F, McConnell T, et al. Costs of fragility hip fractures globally: a systematic review and meta-regression analysis. Osteoporos Int 2017; 28(10):2791–800.
6. Sathiyakumar V, Greenberg SE, Molina CS, et al. Hip fractures are risky business: An analysis of the NSQIP data. Injury 2015;46(4):703–8.
7. Tsang C, Boulton C, Burgon V, et al. Predicting 30-day mortality after hip fracture surgery. Bone Joint Res 2017;6(9):550–6.

8. Garlich JM, Pujari A, Moak Z, et al. Pain Management with Early Regional Anesthesia in Geriatric Hip Fracture Patients. J Am Geriatr Soc 2020;68(9):2043–50.

9. Jones J, Southerland W, Catalani B. The Importance of Optimizing Acute Pain in the Orthopedic Trauma Patient. Orthop Clin North Am 2017;48(4):445–65.

10. Berwin JT, Pearce O, Harries L, et al. Managing polytrauma patients. Injury 2020; 51(10). https://doi.org/10.1016/j.injury.2020.07.051.

11. Jordan RW, Chahal GS, Davies MH. Role of Damage Control Orthopedics and Early Total Care in the Multiple Injured Trauma Patients. Clin Med Insights Trauma Intensive Med 2014;5. https://doi.org/10.4137/cmtim.s12258.

12. Nicholas B, Toth L, Van Wessem K, et al. Borderline femur fracture patients: Early total care or damage control orthopaedics? ANZ J Surg 2011;81(3). https://doi.org/10.1111/j.1445-2197.2010.05582.x.

13. Pape HC, Leenen L. Polytrauma management - What is new and what is true in 2020. J Clin Orthop Trauma 2021;12(1). https://doi.org/10.1016/j.jcot.2020.10.006.

14. Vallier HA, Super DM, Moore TA, et al. Do patients with multiple system injury benefit from early fixation of unstable axial fractures? the effects of timing of surgery on initial hospital course. J Orthop Trauma 2013;27(7). https://doi.org/10.1097/BOT.0b013e3182820eba.

15. Moore TA, Simske NM, Vallier HA. Fracture fixation in the polytrauma patient: Markers that matter. Injury 2020;51:S10–4.

16. Hoehmann CL, Thompson J, Long M, et al. Unnecessary Preoperative Cardiology Evaluation and Transthoracic Echocardiogram Delays Time to Surgery for Geriatric Hip Fractures. J Orthop Trauma 2021;35(4):205–10.

17. Memtsoudis SG. Preoperative Echocardiography in Hip Fracture Patients: A Waste of Time or Good Practice? Anesth Analg 2019;128(2):207–8.

18. Chang JS, Ravi B, Jenkinson RJ, et al. Impact of preoperative echocardiography on surgical delays and outcomes among adults with hip fracture. Bone Joint J 2021;103-B(2):271–8.

19. Nijmeijer WS, Folbert EC, Vermeer M, et al. Prediction of early mortality following hip fracture surgery in frail elderly: The Almelo Hip Fracture Score (AHFS). Injury 2016;47(10):2138–43.

20. Eikelboom R, Gagliardi AR, Gandhi R, et al. Patient and Caregiver Understanding of Prognosis After Hip Fracture. Can Geriatr J 2018;21(3):274–83.

21. Karres J, Kieviet N, Eerenberg J-P, et al. Predicting Early Mortality After Hip Fracture Surgery. J Orthop Trauma 2017;32(1):27–33.

22. Karres J, Heesakkers NA, Ultee JM, et al. Predicting 30-day mortality following hip fracture surgery: Evaluation of six risk prediction models. Injury 2015;46(2):371–7.

23. Kandemir U, Cogan CJ. Preoperative Peripheral Nerve Blocks in Orthopaedic Trauma Surgery: A Guide to Diagnosis-Based Treatment. J Am Acad Orthop Surg 2021;29(19):820–6.

24. Schuijt HJ, Lehmann LS, Javedan H, et al. A Culture Change in Geriatric Traumatology: Holistic and Patient-Tailored Care for Frail Patients with Fractures. J Bone Joint Surg Am 2021;103(18). https://doi.org/10.2106/JBJS.20.02149.

25. Witlox J, Eurelings LSM, De Jonghe JFM, et al. Delirium in elderly patients and the risk of postdischarge mortality, institutionalization, and dementia: A meta-analysis. JAMA 2010;304(4). https://doi.org/10.1001/jama.2010.1013.

26. Castor TD, Meier DE, Levy RN. Ethical aspects of care of the geriatric orthopaedic patient. Clin Orthop Relat Res 1995;316:93–8.

27. Heng M, Eagen CE, Javedan H, et al. Abnormal Mini-Cog is associated with higher risk of complications and delirium in geriatric patients with fracture. J Bone Joint Surg Am 2016;98(9). https://doi.org/10.2106/JBJS.15.00859.

28. Flanagan CD, Joseph NM, Benedick A, et al. Five-year Trends in Opioid Prescribing Following Orthopaedic Trauma. JAAOS Glob Res Rev 2020;4(8). https://doi.org/10.5435/jaaosglobal-d-20-00134.

29. Dada O, Zacarias AG, Ongaigui C, et al. Does rebound pain after peripheral nerve block for orthopedic surgery impact postoperative analgesia and opioid consumption? A narrative review. Int J Environ Res Public Health 2019;16(18). https://doi.org/10.3390/ijerph16183257.

Moving?

Make sure your subscription moves with you!

To notify us of your new address, find your **Clinics Account Number** (located on your mailing label above your name), and contact customer service at:

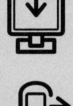

Email: journalscustomerservice-usa@elsevier.com

800-654-2452 (subscribers in the U.S. & Canada)
314-447-8871 (subscribers outside of the U.S. & Canada)

Fax number: 314-447-8029

Elsevier Health Sciences Division
Subscription Customer Service
3251 Riverport Lane
Maryland Heights, MO 63043

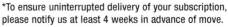